OBSTETRICS AND GYNECOLOGY ADVANCES

AMENORRHEA

OBSTETRICS AND GYNECOLOGY ADVANCES

Additional books in this series can be found on Nova's website
under the Series tab.

Additional e-books in this series can be found on Nova's website
under the eBooks tab.

OBSTETRICS AND GYNECOLOGY ADVANCES

AMENORRHEA

OLIVER CHUKWUJEKWU EZECHI
EDITOR

NOVA BIOMEDICAL

New York

Library of Congress Cataloging-in-Publication Data

ISBN: 978-1-63484-778-0

Library of Congress Control Number: 2016932183

Published by Nova Science Publishers, Inc. † New York

CONTENTS

INTRODUCTION

Amenorrhea is a common presenting complaint of women of reproductive age group. Failure to observe the cyclic monthly menstrual flow is a source of anxiety except for those trying to conceive. The anxiety is unexpected as amenorrhea is seen as a sign of dysfunctional reproductive system.

In order to be a competent practitioner, the trainee and practising physician need not only to acquire a broad knowledge but needs a handy reference material for consultation when they are confronted with challenging case of amenorrhea. In most standard textbooks, because of space constraints various causes of amenorrhea are treated under one or two headings (primary and secondary amenorrhea), making it difficult for the non-specialist physician and trainee to learn the art of managing some relatively uncommon causes.

The purpose of this book is to bridge that gap to provide the trainee and specialist alike with a step by step guide to managing various causes of amenorrhea.

The reader will be able to use the textbook to acquit oneself with the steps involved in the diagnosing and treating a patient with amenorrhea. The aetiology of amenorrhea described in this book is by no means exhaustive but they represent the very common causes of amenorrhea by select group of experienced specialist gynaecologist, researchers and teachers in the field of women's health.

It is recommended that readers of the book follow the chapters sequentially as they are presented, to assist with the learning process. Subjects are mastered by repetition and this book is written in simple english language to enable reader go through the chapters quickly, and when necessary go through them again without getting bored.

I hope that this book will assist you to gain the expertise you so desire. I wish you success on your quest to become a competent expert in the management of amenorrhea.

Oliver Chukwujekwu Ezechi, MD, MPH, PhD, FWACS, FMCOG, FRSPH
Deputy Director Research and Consultant OBGYN
Head, Clinical Sciences Division
Head, Maternal, Reproductive and Child Health Research Group
Nigerian Institute of Medical Research, Lagos Nigeria
Email:oezechi@yahoo.co.uk
April 2016

SECTION I: GENERAL

In: Amenorrhea
Editor: Oliver Chukwujekwu Ezechi

ISBN: 978-1-63484-778-0

Chapter 1

AMENORRHEA: INTRODUCTION, DEFINITIONS AND CLASSIFICATION

Oliver Chukwujekwu Ezechi
Division of Clinical Sciences, Nigerian Institute of Medical Research,
Yaba Lagos, Nigeria

ABSTRACT

Amenorrhea results when the orderly sloughing of the uterine lining on account of the interactions of hormones fails to occur. It elicits anxiety in patients and their family as it suggest abnormality of the reproductive system. The prevalence of amenorrhea not due to physiological states of pregnancy, lactation and menopause ranged from 3-5%, with higher prevalence among athletes. Primary and secondary amenorrhea describes the occurrence of amenorrhea before and after menarche. Identification of abnormal menstrual patterns throughout adolescence may permit early identification of potential health concerns later in life. The majority of the causes of primary and secondary amenorrhea are similar. The common causes are hypothalamic amenorrhea and outflow tract obstruction. Differentiating one cause from the other requires good clinical judgement aided by some investigation.

Keywords: amenorrhea, primary, secondary, pathologic, acquired, congenital

INTRODUCTION

Cyclic menstrual bleeding is an integral part of a woman's experience throughout her reproductive life. Its absence brings mixed feeling for the woman. For the woman trying to have a baby, a welcome development and for the single woman not ready to have a baby, a night mare. For a young girl, failure of menstrual period to appear by age 14-16 years, a source of anxiety for her and her family, warranting consulting a physician. Cessation of menstruation or significant change in menstrual pattern in a hitherto menstruating woman triggers anxiety and a sense of "something is wrong with me." Regular monthly menstruation indicates that the hypothalamo–pituitary–ovarian axis is intact. The hypothalamus, pituitary, and ovaries form an endocrine axis that functions through hormonal regulation and feedback loops. This system governs the regulation of menstruation, which is the cyclic, orderly shedding of the uterine lining [1]. Failure to menstruate between age 14-16 years can be due to a problem at any level of the axis, as can secondary loss of a previously regular cyclical menstruation later in reproductive life. Each woman has her own intrinsic menstrual cycle length during the reproductive years. Regular cycle is established after initial cycle irregularity during the early years of onset of menstruation. The regular rhythm is maintained until the onset of perimenopause in mid- to late forties.

Amenorrhea is the absence or abnormal cessation of spontaneous menstruation in a woman of reproductive age. It is a normal feature in prepubertal, pregnant, lactating and postmenopausal women and should be excluded before diagnosis. Amenorrhea is a symptom, not a disease, and has a variety of causes. Once pregnancy is excluded, the challenge is to determine the exact cause of amenorrhea.

EPIDEMIOLOGY

Amenorrhea, excluding those due to physiological conditions ranged from 5%-20% among women of reproductive age. The prevalence of amenorrhea among the adolescent females was found to be higher than the general population [2]. The frequency of amenorrhea was reported to be 5% in Mexico [3] and Nigeria [4], 8-13% in Venezuela [5-7] and 20% in India [8]. In a study conducted in USA and Canada by Souza and colleagues, amenorrhea was found in about two-third of women in one form of exercise [9]. HIV infection impact on burden of amenorrhea. A study from Lagos Nigeria among HIV positive women showed that HIV-positive women experienced more menstrual abnormalities of amenorrhea, oligomenorrhoea, and irregular periods compared to their HIV-negative controls. Amenorrhea was found in 3.8% of the HIV positive women compared to 1.8% among the HIV negative women [10].

PATHOPHYSIOLOGY

Menstrual cycle is an orderly progression of coordinated hormonal events that stimulates growth of a follicle to release an egg and prepare the uterine lining for embryo in readiness for implantation. Failure of the released egg from the ovary to fertilise and form an embryo causes drop in the level of hormones of pregnancy that maintain the endometrium. Subsequently, the decidua of the endometrium sloughs off as menstrual flow in preparation for another cycle.

Normal female chromosomal pattern (46 XX), intact and coordinated hypothalamo–pituitary–ovarian axis, patent outflow tract, responsive endometrium and functioning thyroid and adrenal glands are essential for the onset and continuation of normal menstruation. Dysfunction in any of the above may result in failure of initiation or continuation of menstruation.

DEFINITIONS AND CLASSIFICATION

Several factors are known to cause amenorrhea making a simple classification difficult. Amenorrhea is traditional classified as either primary or secondary. The distinction is artificial and descriptive as the same condition may be responsible for both primary and secondary amenorrhea. Unfortunately the classification is the most commonly used, as it has some practical clinical value of given clue to the cause of amenorrhea and outcome of management. While secondary amenorrhea is more likely to result from acquired disease, generally more amenable to treatment, and has a better prognosis, primary amenorrhea are often due to either a genetic or gross developmental abnormality of the ovarian or müllerian structures. It is more difficult to manage and with poorer prognosis. Amenorrhea has also been classified as physiologic or pathologic, or based on the compartments of the hypothalamo–pituitary–ovarian axis where the problem occurs (Figure 1).

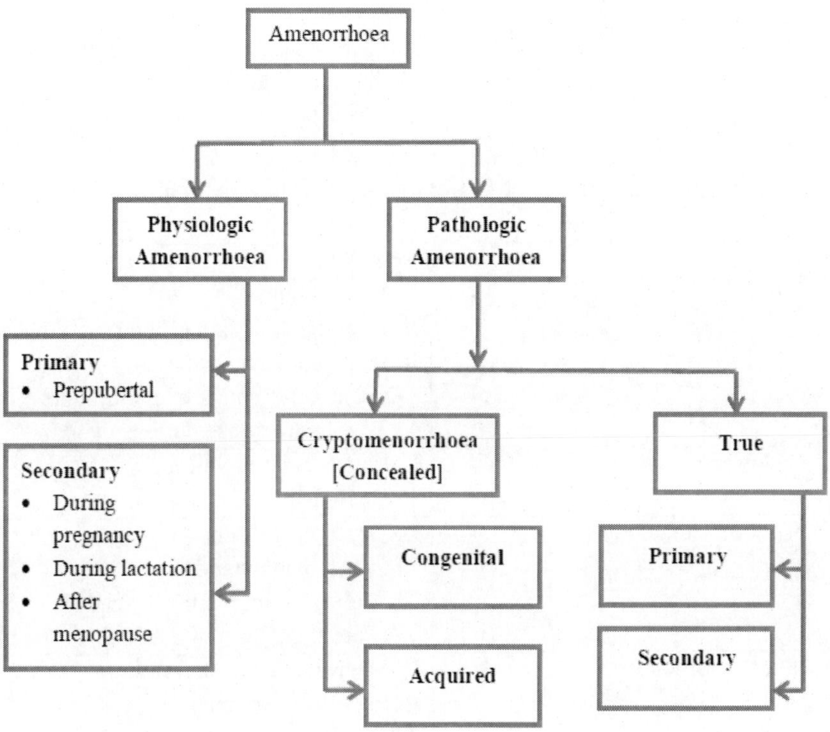

Figure 1. Classification of amenorrhea.

Physiologic Amenorrhea

The occurrence of amenorrhea is said to be normal in four states, before puberty, during pregnancy, during lactation and after menopause. Before puberty the pituitary gonadotropins are not adequate enough to stimulate the ovary for effective production of oestrogen. The low level of oestrogen during this period is insufficient to cause uterine endometrial bleeding. The duration of amenorrhea in breastfeeding women is highly variable, even among similar groups with comparable breastfeeding practices. The observed difference is due to the natural variation in sensitivity of the breast-hypothalamus-pituitary system to suckling in individual women and the quality of the suckling stimulus.

Pathologic Amenorrhea

This type of amenorrhea is due to an organic disease; which could be anatomical or functional. It could further be classified as congenital e.g., Kallmann syndrome, testicular feminisation or acquired type as in Ashermans or Sheehan's syndrome. Pathologic amenorrhea could be concealed as in imperforate hymen or true as in chronic anovulation.

Primary Amenorrhea

The failure to initiate menstruation by age 16 years, in the presence of normal growth and secondary sexual characteristics, by age of 14 year, in the absence of secondary sexual characteristics. The causes of primary amenorrhea are group into eight categories (Table 1).

Table 1. Causes of Primary amenorrhea by group

Group	Specific causes
A. Hypogonadotropic hypogonadism	I. Delayed puberty II. Hypothalamic and pituitary dysfunction III. Kallmann syndrome IV. Central nervous system tumours V. 17 α hydroxylase deficiency
B. Hypergonadotropic hypogonadism	I. Primary ovarian failure II. Resistance ovarian syndrome
C. Abnormal chromosomal pattern	I. Turner's syndrome II. Pure gonadal dysgenesis III. Androgen insensitivity syndrome IV. Partial deletion of the X chromosome
D. Outflow tract abnormality	I. Transverse vaginal system II. Imperforate hymen III. Vaginal and cervical atresia IV. Absence of the uterus
E. Thyroid and adrenal dysfunction	I. Adrenogenital syndrome II. Cretinism
F. Metabolic disorder	I. Obesity II. Juvenile diabetes

Secondary Amenorrhea

The absence of menstruation for 6 months in a woman that has previous established normal menstruation. However, some authorities consider three or four months of amenorrhea as the cut off limit. Secondary amenorrhea is generally categories as concealed and true secondary amenorrhea. Its causes are further grouped into categories depending on the aetiology (Table 2).

Table 2. Causes of secondary amenorrhea

Group	Specific cause(s)
A. Vaginal	i. Labial agglutination ii. Vaginal atresia following genital mutilation iii. Insertion of corrosive into the vagina
B. Uterine	i. Tuberculosis ii. Radiation iii. Asherman's syndrome iv. Surgical ablation
C. Ovarian	i. Premature ovarian failure ii. Polycystic ovarian syndrome iii. Resistant ovarian syndrome iv. Feminising ovarian tumours
D. Pituitary	i. Sheehan's Syndrome ii. Prolactinoma iii. Simmonds disease
E. Hypothalamus	i. Carniopharyngioma ii. Anorexia nervosa iii. Trauma
F. Adrenal gland	i. Cushing syndrome
G. Thyroid gland	i. Hyprothyroidism
H. Drugs	i. Pyschotropic drugs ii. Antihypertensive drugs
I. Systemic illness	i. Infections: HIV, Tuberculosis and toxoplasmosis ii. Anorexia nervosa iii. Malnutrition iv. Severe anaemia

CONCLUSION

Amenorrhea is a common finding in gynaecology practice. The common causes are hyperprolactinaemia, hypothalamic amenorrhea, Ashermans syndrome and polycystic ovarian syndrome. Differentiating one cause from the other requires by good clinical judgement aided some investigation.

REFERENCES

[1] Harlow S D, Ephross SA. Epidemiology of menstruation and its relevance to women's health. *Epidemiologic Reviews* 1995; 17(2): 265-286.

[2] Harlow SD, Campbell OM. Epidemiology of menstrual disorders in developing countries: a systematic review. *BJOG: An International Journal of Obstetrics and Gynaecology* 12005;11(1): 6-16.

[3] Hernandez I, Cervera-Aguilar R, Verdara MD, Ayala AR. Prevalence and etiology of secondary amenorrhea in a selected Mexican population. *Ginecol Obstet Mex* 1999;67: 374-376.

[4] Ikechebelu, JI. Prevalence of gynaecological diseases in Nnewi. Nigeria. *Nig. J Clin Pract*, 2005;556, 8.

[5] Nun˜ez Troconis J, Amesty N, Sandoval J. Trastornos menstruales en estudiantes universitarias (Menstrual disorders in college students). Amenorrea y Oligomenorrea (Amenorrhea and Oligomenorrhea). *Rev Obstet Ginecol Venez* 1990;50:138-141.

[6] Nun˜ez Troconis J, Amesty N, Sandoval J. Trastornos menstruales en estudiantes universitarias (Menstrual disorders in college students. Amenorrhea and Oligomenorrhea). II Menarquia y dismenorrea (II menarche and dysmenorrhea). *Rev Obstet Ginecol Venez* 1991;51:105-108.

[7] Nun˜ez Troconis J, Giro´n Pa´ez H, Nun˜ez Virla L. Alteraciones del ciclo menstrual en internas y residents (Menstrual abnormalities in internal and residents). *Rev Obstet Ginecol Venez* 1999; 59:257-262.

[8] Bang RA, Bang AT, Baitule M, Choudhary Y, Sarmukaddam S, Tale O. High prevalence of gynaecological diseases in rural Indian women. *Lancet* 1989;1:85-88.

[9] De Souza, M. J., Toombs, R. J., Scheid, J. L., O'Donnell, E., West, S. L., and Williams, N. I. High prevalence of subtle and severe menstrual disturbances in exercising women: confirmation using daily hormone measures. *Human reproduction*, 2010;25(2), 491-503.

[10] Ezechi, O. C., Jogo, A., Gab-Okafor, C., Onwujekwe, D. I., Ezeobi, P. M., Gbajabiamila, T. et al. Effect of HIV-1 infection and increasing immunosuppression on menstrual function. *Journal of Obstetrics and Gynaecology Research*, 2010;36(5), 1053-1058.

[11] Speroff L, Fritz MA. Clinical Gynecologic Endocrinology and Infertility. Lippincott, Williams and Wilkins (2005). p. 403.

In: Amenorrhea
Editor: Oliver Chukwujekwu Ezechi
ISBN: 978-1-63484-778-0

Chapter 2

MENSTRUAL PHYSIOLOGY AND ABNORMALITIES

Endurance Ediriverere Aghahowa and Oliver Chukwujekwu Ezechi
Division of Clinical Sciences, Nigerian Institute of Medical Research,
Lagos, Nigeria

ABSTRACT

Menstruation marks the beginning of the process by which the uterus, prepares itself for pregnancy. Each month the uterine endometrium is shed, producing a period and a new lining is grown to replace it. The onset of the first menstruation occurs at puberty, termed menarche and its cessation, termed the menopause. Menstrual cycle is the repetitive monthly change that occurs in the ovaries and the endometrium of the uterus in human females of reproductive age. A normal menstrual cycle varies from 21-35 days with a mean of 28 days. However, it is only about 12.4% of women that have a 28 day cycle. The variations in normal menstrual cycle among women is attributable to the variation in woman's age, nutrition, weight, level of physical activities, level of stress and even genetics. Menstrual cycle is dependent on the complex interplay of four key hormones: oestrogen and progesterone released from the ovaries, Follicle Stimulating and Leuitinising Hormones released by pituitary gland. During the menstrual cycle, cyclical changes occur simultaneously in the ovaries and uterus and are termed ovarian and uterine cycle respectively. Understanding the complex interplay of the hypothalamic – pituitary-ovarian axis and its feedback loops and the resultant effects on the female reproductive organs provides a foundation for family planning, management of infertility and menstrual abnormalities. Pathological changes or conditions could result in abnormalities of the menstrual cycle.

INTRODUCTION

Normal menstrual function depends on the complex interaction between the hypothalamic–pituitary–ovarian axis and endogenous hormones. Every month the uterine endometrium is shed, producing a menstrual period and a new lining is grown to replace it. The onset of the first menstruation occurs at puberty, termed menarche and its cessation, termed the menopause. Menstrual cycle is the repetitive monthly change that occurs in the ovaries and the endometrium of the uterus in human females of reproductive age. A normal menstrual cycle varies from 21-35 days with a mean of 28 days. Even though most women will claim regular menstrual cycle, only 12.4% have a 28 day cycle. The variations in normal menstrual cycle among women is attributable to the variation in woman's age, nutrition, weight, level of physical activities, level of stress and even genetics [1].

Menstrual cycle is dependent on the complex interplay of four key hormones, oestrogen and progesterone released from the ovaries, Follicle Stimulating and Leuitinising Hormones released by pituitary gland. Menstrual abnormalities results from the alteration in these hormones. Women with abnormal menstrual cycles may have a higher risk of cardiovascular disease, type 2 diabetes, osteoporosis, infertility, and breast and endometrial cancers [1, 2].

Although it is known that modifiable lifestyle behaviour affects normal menstrual cycle function, the underlying mechanisms connecting lifestyle factors to menstrual function are unclear, but are likely due to alterations in hormonal patterns. The alteration in hormone pattern in turn predicts the occurrence and timing of ovulation and growth of the endometrial lining [2, 3].

Understanding the interplay of the hypothalamic –pituitary-ovarian axis and its feedback loops and the resultant effects on the female reproductive organs, the ovaries and the uterus provides a foundation for the management of menstrual cycle abnormalities.

Normal Menstrual Cycle

During the menstrual cycle, cyclical changes occur simultaneously in both the ovaries and the uterus and are termed ovarian and uterine cycle respectively [1-4].

Ovarian Cycle

The ovarian cycle has 3 phases of follicular, luteal and ovulation that separate them. Both follicular and luteal phases last on the average 14 days each. While the luteal phase last about 14 days without great variation, the variation noticed in menstrual cycle is due to the variation in follicular phase of the ovarian cycle.

In the first few days of the follicular phase of the menstrual cycle, low levels of estrogen, progesterone and inhibin creates a positive feedback on the hypothalamus leading to the release of Gondadotrophin Releasing Hormone (GnRH) and subsequent release of Follicle Stimulating Hormone (FSH) and Luteinizing hormone (LH). But the increase in FSH is slightly higher and precedes the increase in LH by few days.

Follicular phase as the name implies is dominated by follicular growth. Primordial follicles which consist of a single layer of granulosa cells and an ovum experiences an increase in number of layers of the granulosa cells and an increase in size of the ovum to become primary follicles. A cohort of primary follicles [6-12] are stimulated at the beginning of each menstrual cycle. The primary follicle further develops to become antral follicle (presence of an antrum – accumulation of follicular fluids secreted by granulosa cells). The antral vesicles grow to become vesicular follicles.

Follicle stimulating hormone (FSH) stimulates the production of estrogen by the granulosa cells. While LH stimulates the theca interna cells (the inner layer of the capsule of the follicle) to produce androgens which are converted (aromatized) to estradiol which is a form of estrogen in the granulosa cells, under the influence of FSH.

The secreted estrogen causes the granulosa cells to form increased number of FSH receptors and become more sensitive to FSH leading to further stimulation of the follicle and greater levels of estrogen secretion (positive feedback). Both FSH and estrogen promotes LH receptors on the granulosa cells creating further increase in follicular secretions by the activities of the theca interna cells. By mid-follicular phase, there is higher levels of estradiol/ estrogens, increased FSH and LH receptors. A high level of estradiol exerts a negative feedback on the anterior pituitary to suppress further secretion of FSH.

Interestingly, of the 6-12 follicles, only one becomes fully matured. It outgrows the others to become the dominate follicle while the others become atretic. It has been postulated that the follicle with the highest concentration of LH receptors becomes the dominant follicle as it responds more to the increasing levels of LH and generates more estradiol for increased growth of its follicular cells while those with less receptors become atretic in the presence of declining FSH levels. As Estradiol levels rises, it reaches a peak that triggers the LH surge from the anterior pituitary by a positive feedback mechanism. This surge occurs about 24-36 hours before ovulation. A high level of LH inhibits estradiol production and it also converts both the granulosa and theca cells into progesterone secreting cells. Preovulatory, there is a drop in estradiol and a small rise in progesterone. LH surge also induces the resumption of oocyte meiotic maturation.

Under the influence of LH activities, proteolytic enzymes such as plasminogen activator and plasmin are released from the theca externa (outer layer of the capsule of the follicle). These enzymes act on the follicular wall to dissolve it resulting in a weakening of the follicular capsule. LH surge also results in an increase in follicular blood flow and an inflammatory type response with production of vasodilatory prostalglandins causing dissolution and weakening of wall of the follicular capsule. A weakened wall in the presence of increased volume of the follicle and other factors lead to follicle rupture and release of the ovum. This process by which the ovum is released from the graafian follicle (matured ovarian follicle) is termed ovulation.

After the release of the ovum, the remaining granulosa and theca cells becomes filled with yellow pigment and lipids by a process called leutinization and form the corpus luteum. The Corpus luteum secretes both progesterone and estrogen but higher levels of progesterone. Rising levels of these sex hormones exert a negative feedback on the hypothalamus and anterior pituitary to inhibit secretion of LH and FSH. This prevents new follicular maturation during the luteal phase.

In the absence of fertilisation, the matured corpus luteum which has become less sensitive to LH loses its secretory ability at about 10-12 days to become corpus albicans with a resultant decline in progesterone and estrogen. Withdrawal of these sex hormones (progesterone which has a stabilising effect on the uterine endometrium) will lead to spasm of endometrial blood vessels, shedding of the endometrium which culminates as menstruation. Low levels of the sex hormones and inhibin results in a loss of the negative feedback effect on FSH and LH secretion. The anterior pituitary resumes its secretion of FSH and LH and ushers in a new ovarian cycle.

Uterine Cycle

As the ovary and ovum undergoes changes during the ovarian cycle; the uterine endometrium also undergoes various changes as a result of variations in the levels of LH and FSH. The hormones oestradiol and progesterone induces changes on the endometrium resulting in three distinguishable phases of the uterine cycle - menstrual, proliferative and secretory phases.

The menstrual phase of the uterine cycle begins at the end of 28 days in the absence of fertilisation. In the absence of fertilisation, the corpus luteum involutes and the supply of both sex hormones decline and the support for endometrial growth is lost. This results in reduction in endometrial thickness. Involution causes a release of vasoconstrictive prostaglandins which leads to hypoxia and subsequent necrosis of the upper layer of the endometrium which becomes desquamated and is shed and expel through the vaginal as blood and is seen as a visible evidence of the menstrual cycle- menstruation. This marks day 1 of a new menstrual cycle. Vaginal bleeding last about 5-6 days and ceases as the endometrium enters proliferative phase and regenerates.

Post menstruation shedding of the endometrium leaves behind a single layered endometrium. Under the influence of estrogen as noted at the beginning of the ovarian cycle, the cells of the uterine endometrium proliferate rapidly with re-epitheliazation, revascularisation, growth of new glands and increased number of stromal cells increasing its thickness rom 0.5 mm post menstruation to about 3.5-5.5 mm thick [5].

Under the influence of estrogen, the cervical glands secrete a less thick mucus that lines the cervical canal. The secretions has increased water content and become more fluid. This serves as a favourable medium for sperm transport through the cervical canal. This stringy mucus may be noticed by women as a monitoring indicator for ovulation. The end of the proliferative phase coincides with the ovulation at day 14 in a 28 day cycle.

Secretory phase of uterine cycle occurs after ovulation. In this phase of the cycle there is an increased level of progesterone than estrogens. This reduces the influence of estrogen on the uterine endometrium. Progesterone induces further growth in the endometrial glands which becomes tortous and secretes a clear fluid; there is rapid growth of blood vessels and vasodilation; increased secretion and storage of glycogen and lipids in endometrial stromal cells. This phase prepares the uterus for implantation of a fertilized ovum. This phase lasts for about 14 days. However, if fertilization does not occur, the uterus enters the menstrual phase to begin a new menstrual cycle.

Menstrual Cycle Length

The length of the menstrual cycle is counted from the first day of menstruation to the day before the next menstrual flow. This first day in the most recent menstrual flow is termed the last menstrual period (LMP). The mean length of menstrual cycle is 28 days, however only about 12.4% of women have a 28 days cycle [6, 7]. There are variations in most women from 21 to 35 days attributable to varying factors such as a woman's age, nutrition, weight, level of physical activities, stress and genetics. Average duration of menstrual blood flow is 5-7 days. While average volume of menstrual blood loss is 35-50 mls without significant clots but about 10% of women experiences losses of over 80 mls/cycle [8].

A variation in menstrual length occurs in the follicular phase rather than the luteal phase which remains relatively constant [4]. This variation is thought to be due to follicle selection where there is competition between oocytes to become the primary oocyte. Lifestyle such as smoking and exercise has also been attributed [9, 10].

Fertile Period

Fertile period is the days in the menstrual cycle when the potential for achieving conception is highest. This is usually considered to be 5 days before ovulation and 24 hours after ovulation. This 6 days calculation, takes into account the 5 days average lifespan of a sperm in the female reproductive tract and the 24 hour lifespan of the egg after ovulation. For a 28 day cycle length, ovulation occurs on the 14th day thus fertile period is from day 8 to day 15.

However, since majority of women do not have a 28 day cycle, a method of calculating fertile period was derived. This is the calendar method. The calculations are based on at least 6 previous menstrual cycles which are documented. The shortest and longest cycles are noted. The subtraction of 20 from the shortest cycle gives the first day of the fertile period and subtracting 11 from the longest cycle gives the last day of the fertile period. For example, if the shortest cycle is 29 days and the longest cycle 35 days, 29 minus 20 will give day 9 while 35-11 will give day 24, the fertile period is likely to be days 9 to 24 of her menstrual cycle. However considering the fact that variations often occur in the menstrual cycle length, a simple method was developed known as the standard day's method. It simply states that the fertile time in a woman with between 28 and 32 days cycle length is days 8 to 19 of the menstrual cycle [8].

Monitoring Ovulation Time

Pregnancy is the ultimate evidence of ovulation, However since ovulation cannot be monitored posthoc, some indicators of ovulation have been derived from physiologic changes that occur within the menstrual cycle. These indicators are:

Changes in basal body temperature (BBT): Progesterone causes an increase in basal body temperature. The increase in progesterone levels immediately after ovulation causes a temperature rise by least 0.2 degree Celsius [9].

Cervical secretions: Under the influence of rising levels of estrogen, the glands of the cervix secrete mucus that lines the cervical canal. The mucus is thinner and stringy or stretchier. The rising levels of estrogen alter the cervical secretions from being thick and sticky to becoming gradually more transparent, wetter, and stretchier. The secretions become more fluid because of increased water content. The sperm move easily in these fertile secretions, which facilitate their movement upwards through the genital tract.

Cervical position: Both sex hormones estrogen and progesterone has effects on the connective tissue and muscular structure of the cervix. By gently palpating, the woman notes the position, the consistency and cervical os whether open or closed. When the cervix is high, soft and open, it is fertile period until the cervix becomes low, firm and closed for at least 3 days [9].

Mittelschmerz Pain: This is a one sided lower abdominal pain that occurs at or around ovulation. This pain could occur as a result of the increased size of the follicle which stretches the surface of the ovary. It could also be attributable to irritation of the lining of the abdomen by the fluid released from the ruptured egg follicle during ovulation. This pain is usually mild and occurs in few of women.

Other Indicators: Increased libido and a heightened sense of smell have been reported in some women some days before ovulation.

Menstrual Abnormalities

In determining if a menstrual cycle is abnormal, four basic parameters are used to define the bleeding component of the menstrual experience. These are:

- Regularity of onset (predictable onset with respect to date
- Frequency of onset (e.g., every 28 days)
- Duration of menstrual flow (e.g., 5 days in duration)
- Heaviness (or volume) of menstrual flow

The "normal" limits for menstrual parameters in the reproductive years are shown in Table 1.

It is known that certain pathologic conditions and stressful situations can affect a woman's menstrual cycle. The abnormalities of the menstrual cycle include amenorrhea, intermenstrual bleeding, dysmenorrhoea and abnormal uterine bleeding (AUB). While amenorrhea and intermenstrual bleed is discussed in the other chapters, dysmenorrhoea and AUB will be discussed in this chapter.

Table 1. FIGO recommendation for normal limits of menstrual dimensions

Clinical dimensions of menstruation and the menstrual cycle	Descriptive terms	Normal limits (5th to 95th percentiles)
Frequency of menses (days)	Frequent	<24
	Normal	24-38
	Infrequent	>38
Regularity of menses (cycle to cycle variation over 12 months)	Absent	No bleeding
	Regular	Variation + or - 2 to 20 days
	Irregular	Variation >20 days
Duration of flow (days)	Prolonged	>8.0 days
	Normal	4.5-8.0 days
	Shortened	<4.5 days
Volume of monthly blood loss (mL)	Heavy	>80
	Normal	5-80
	Light	<5

Dysmenorrhoea

Ideally menstruation should be relatively painless, and often associated with cramps in ovulating women. The cramp usually resolves spontaneously and does not interfere with daily activities. In dysmenorrhoea, the menstrual pain is of sufficient magnitude as to incapacitate day to day activities. Dysmenorrhoea is commonly classified as either primary or secondary types.

Primary dysmenorrhoea: Painful menstruation without an identifiable pathology. It occurs about 6 months after menarche when ovulatory cycles have begun. However, it may set in with the first menstrual flow at menarche. The mechanism of the initiation of uterine pain in primary dysmenorrhoea is not clearly known, however available evidence do suggest that prostaglandin $PGF_{2\alpha}$ synthesis and release play a central role. The released $PGF_{2\alpha}$ is a strong vasoconstrictor, which causes ischaemia of the uterine muscle causing pain. Prostaglandins also causes the release of endothelins, leukotrienes and platelet activating factor which are vasoconstrictors and stimulate uterine muscle contractions, and ultimately pain [19, 20]. Imbalance in the autonomic nervous control of uterine muscles, abnormal anatomical and functional uterine muscles and psychosomatic factors are other possible mechanisms of initiation of uterine pain in primary dysmenorrhea.

Primary dysmenorrhoea is mainly a problem in adolescent girls and usually appears within 2 years of the first menstrual flow. Adolescent from wealthy homes are mostly at risk and there may be a history of dysmenorrhoea in the nuclear family.

Dysmenorrhoeic pain starts a few hours before the onset of menstruation and rarely last for more than 2 days. The pain is spasmodic and confined to lower abdomen and last for few hours.

The majority of the patients can successfully be managed with explanation and assurance. Analgesic and antispasmodic drugs are useful in mild cases. Encouragement of normal activities and emptying of bowel may be useful. In severe cases prostaglandin synthetase inhibitors, oral contraceptive pills and dydrogesterone have been used with good result. Any of the surgical treatment option (Table 2) can be deplored if medical treatment fails and laparoscopy excludes pelvic pathology.

Secondary dysmenorrhoea: Painful menstruation in the presence of an identifiable pelvic pathology. Causes include pelvic inflammatory disease, uterine fibroid, ovarian cysts, intra uterine device and endometriosis (Table 3).

Patients with secondary dysmenorrhoea presents with dull back and lower abdominal pain. It starts 3-5 days before the menses and is relieved with the start of flow. The onset and duration of the pain is related to the pathology. Unlike in primary dysmenorrhoea, there is no systemic discomfort.

The primary goal of treatment of secondary dysmenorrhoea is targeted at removing the offending pathology.

Table 2. Surgical option for treating primary dysmenorrhea

1. Transcutaneous electrical nerve stimulation
2. Dilatation of cervical canal
3. Laparoscopic uterine nerve stimulation
4. Laparoscopic presacral neurectomy

Table 3. Common causes of secondary dysmenorrhoea

1. Cervical stenosis
2. Chronic pelvic infection
3. Endometrial polyp
4. Uterine fibroid
5. Intrauterine contraceptive device (IUCD)
6. Endometriosis
7. Pelvic adhesions
8. Obstruction due to Müllerian abnormality
9. Fixed retroversion of the uterus

Membranous dysmenorrhea is rare type of dysmenorrhoea. It causes intense cramping pain as a result of the passage of the intact endometrial cast through an undilated cervix [13].

Abnormal Uterine Bleeding

The uterus sheds a limited amount of blood (less than 80 ml) every 28 days for a duration lasting not more than 8 days. Uterine bleeding that occurs erratically or excessive regular menstrual bleeding is considered to be abnormal uterine bleeding. Once a woman who is not taking hormone therapy enters menopause and the menstrual cycles have ended, any uterine bleeding is considered abnormal.

Abnormal uterine bleeding (AUB) is an extremely common clinical problem that affect over one-fifth of premenopausal women above 35 years of age. AUB has been shown to be the fourth most common gynaecologic reason for hospital admission in the United States of America [13]. It is reported that heavy bleeders lose about 4 working weeks yearly which impact on family income and national development [13].

Until recently, the terms and terminology used in identifying various abnormalities in menstrual frequency, duration of flow, regularity and volume were confusing and often ambiguous. The terminologies were English language derivatives of Latin and Greek root words which poorly defined, creating ambiguity in meaning and usage. Experts in the field of women's health in 2005, recommended the discarding of confusing terminology with a simple descriptive terms that could be understood by patients and easily translated into other languages. This recommendation resulted in the "The PALM-COEIN Classification System" created by the Federation International Gynecology Obstetrics (FIGO) Menstrual Disorders Group and adopted in 2009, FIGO World Congress of Gynecology and Obstetrics [14].

The PALM-COEIN Classification System

A new FIGO classification system for causes of abnormal uterine bleeding in non-gravid women of reproductive age. The classification system accepted as FIGO classification in 2010. In this classification system the term amenorrhea was retained but other confusing and ambiguous terminologies were discarded (Table 4).

Table 4. Discarded Terminologies in Palm Coein classification

Menorrhagia	Hypermenorrhea	Hypomenorrhea
Menometrorrhagia	Polymenorrhea	Polymenorrhagia
Epimenorrhea	Epimenorrhagia	Uterine hemorrhage
Dysfunctional uterine bleeding	Functional uterine bleeding	Metropathica hemorrhagica
Oligomenorrhea		

The recommended terminology, definitions, and classifications of symptoms of AUB are detailed in this section.

Disturbances of Regularity

- Irregular Menstrual Bleeding: Bleeding of >20 days in individual cycle lengths over a period of one year.
- Absent Menstrual Bleeding (amenorrhea): No bleeding in a 90-day period.

Disturbances in Frequency

- Infrequent Menstrual Bleeding: One or two episodes in a 90-day period.
- Frequent Menstrual Bleeding: More than four episodes in a 90-day period.

Disturbances of Heaviness of Flow

- Heavy Menstrual Bleeding: Excessive menstrual blood loss that interferes with the woman's physical, emotional, social, and material quality of life and can occur alone or in combination with other symptoms.
- Heavy and Prolonged Menstrual Bleeding: Less common than heavy menstrual bleeding (HMB). It is important to make a distinction from HMB given they may have different etiologies and respond to different therapies.
- Light Menstrual Bleeding: Based on patient complaint, rarely related to pathology.

Disturbance of the Duration of Flow

- Prolonged Menstrual Bleeding: Menstrual periods exceeding 8 days in duration on a regular basis.
- Shortened Menstrual Bleeding: Uncommon, defined as bleeding of no longer than 2 days.
- Irregular Non menstrual Bleeding: Irregular episodes of bleeding, often light and short, occurring between normal menstrual periods. Mostly associated with benign or malignant structural lesions. May occur during or following sexual intercourse.

Bleeding Outside Reproductive Age

- Postmenopausal Bleeding: Bleeding occurring >1 year after the acknowledged menopause.
- Precocious Menstruation: Usually associated with other signs of precocious puberty, occurring before 9 years of age.

Acute AUB: An episode of heavy bleeding that, in the opinion of the clinician, is of sufficient quantity to require immediate intervention to prevent further blood loss. Acute AUB may present in the context of existing chronic AUB or might occur without such a history. Although women of reproductive age with acute AUB require immediate intervention, their follow-up may be largely dependent upon whether they require investigation and ongoing care for an underlying chronic condition [13, 14].

Visually objective structural criteria	
P	Polyps (AUB-P)
A	Adenomyosis (AUB-A)
L	Leiomyoma (AUB-L) → Submucosa / Other
M	Malignancy (AUB-M)

Unrelated to structural anomalies/ Entities not yet defined	
C	Coagulopathy (AUB-C)
O	Ovulatory disorders (AUB-O)
E	Endometrial (AUB-E)
I	Iatrogenic (AUB-I)
N	Not Classified

Leiomyoma sub classification system		
SM - Submucous	0	pedunculated intra-cavitary
	1	< 50% Intramural
	2	≥ 50% intramural
	3	Contacts endometrium; 100% intramural
	4	Intramural
	5	Subserous ≥ 50% intramural
	6	Subserous < 50% intramural
	7	Subserous pedunculated
	8	Other (specify e.g. cervical, parasitic)
Hybrid Leiomyoma (impact both endometrium and serosa	Two numbers are listed separated by a hyphen. By convention, the first refers to the relationship with endometrium. While the second refers to the relationship to the serosa. One e.g. below	
	2-5	Submucous and Subserous, each with less than half the diameter in the endometrial and peritoneal cavities respectively

Figure 1. Causes of abnormal uterine bleeding according to FIGO Palm Coein classification 2010.

Chronic AUB: Bleeding from the uterine corpus that is abnormal in volume, regularity, and/or timing, and has been present for the majority of the past 6 months. Chronic AUB would not, in the opinion of the clinician, require immediate intervention [13, 14].

Intermenstrual bleeding (IMB): Bleeding occurring between clearly defined cyclic and predictable menses. Such bleeding may occur at random times or may manifest in a predictable fashion at the same day in each cycle. This designation is designed to replace the word "metrorrhagia," which has been abandoned by the new classification [13, 14].

Patterns of Bleeding: The "shape" of the volume of the bleeding pattern over the days of one menstrual period. It is usually recognized that about 90% of the total menstrual flow is lost within the first 3 days of the cycle, with day 1 or 2 the heaviest. In women with AUB this pattern is variable [13, 14].

In the Palm Coein classification, the basic system comprises of four categories that are defined by visually objective structural criteria (PALM—Polyp, Adenomyosis, Leiomyoma, and Malignancy or hyperplasia); four (COEI – Coagulopathy, Ovulatory dysfunction, Endometrial, Iatrogenic) that are unrelated to structural anomalies; and one (N) reserved for entities that are not yet classified (Figure 1).

The leiomyoma category (L) is secondarily subdivided into those patients who have at least one submucous myoma (L_{SM}) and those with myomas that do not impact the endometrial cavity (L_o). Further subclassification of the SM group is according to the Wamsteker system [14, 15], with added categorizations for the intramural, subserous, and transmural lesions.

Causes of Abnormal Uterine Bleeding

The causes of abnormal uterine bleeding according to Palm coein classification (Figure 1) is discussed below [13, 14, 16].

1. Polyps (AUB-P): The most common presenting symptom is abnormal vaginal bleeding. Polyp accounts for all causes of abnormal vaginal bleeding in about 39% of pre-menopausal and 25% in post-menopausal women. In the PC classification it is categorized as either present or absent. Ultrasound scan especially transvaginal USS, saline infusion sonography, and hysteroscopy are used for diagnosis of polyp.
2. Adenomyosis (AUB-A): Over two-third of women with adenomyosis presents with symptoms of AUB. The remaining one third presents with dysmenorrhea. Only less than one-fifth of women diagnosed with adenomyosis present with both AUB and dysmenorrhoea. Ultrasound or MRI is used for diagnosis.
3. Leiomyomas (AUB-L_{SM} or AUB-L_O): Commonly known as uterine fibroid. It is the most common benign tumor of the genital tract. Over 60% of women above 45 years of age have leiomyomas. Women with submucosal leiomyoma present more frequently with AUB compared to those with intramural and subserosal leiomyomas.
4. Malignancy (AUB-M): The main symptom of endometrial neoplasia is AUB. However over two-third of post-menopausal bleeding has benign cause. Other causes of postmenopausal bleeding are endometrial hyperplasia (15%) and endometrial cancer (15%). This category of AUB includes both premalignant and malignant lesions. About half of patients with endometrial hyperplasia also have concurrent carcinoma.

5. Coagulopathies (AUB-C): Available evidence shows that between 10-15% of women with heavy menstrual bleeding have haemostatic disorders. This is often overlooked during investigation for AUB.
6. Ovulatory Dysfunction (AUB-O): Most cases of unpredictable menstrual cycle with variable flow are associated with diseases of endocrine gland (e.g., hypothyroidism or polycyctic ovary disease. In management of patients with AUB, evaluation of possible causes of anovulation should be investigated.
7. Endometrial Causes (AUB-E): Patients in this category often present with heavy menstrual bleeding or intermenstrual bleeding. Regular cycles, normal ovulation and no definable cause of AUB is the norm rather than the exception.
8. Iatrogenic (AUB-I): Intrauterine contraceptive device, steroids and drug that affect ovulation or coagulation are some of the causes. Treatment is to remove the offending agent.
9. Not Yet Classified (AUB-N): This category is reserved for entities that are poorly defined and/or not well examined. As evidence emerges, conditions under this category will be moved to other categories.

Notation of AUB

In some cases of AUB, the woman may be found to have more than one potential entity contributing to symptoms of AUB. A notation approach has been designed to enable categorization. For example, if a patient with AUB is found to have leiomyoma, polyp and on intrauterine contraceptive device, she would be categorized as follows: AUB P_1 A_0 L_1 M_0 – C_0 O_0 E_0 I_1 N_0. This may be abbreviated as: AUB – P; L; I.

Evaluation of Abnormal Uterine Bleeding

History: Evaluation of AUB should begin with a historic review of patient's symptomatology; including treatment history. Attending physician should determine the age of menarche and menopause, menstrual bleeding patterns and severity of bleeding (clots or flooding). Enquire of the duration and amount of bleeding; factors that seem to bring the bleeding on; symptoms that occur along with the bleeding such as pain, fever, or vaginal odour. Any relationship of the bleeding to sexual intercourse. Any personal or family history of bleeding disorders. The woman's medical history and medications she is taking.

Physical examination: During physical examination the physician should assess the overall health of the woman. Pelvic examination should be conducted to confirm that the bleeding is from the uterus and other sites outside the uterus. Physician should look out for any obvious lesions, determine the size and shape of the uterus and signs of cervical bleeding. It is important to conduct cervical cancer screening.

Laboratory investigation: In the investigation of women with AUB some test should always be conducted as a basic minimum (Table 5).

Table 5. Basic test in determine the cause of abnormal uterine bleeding

Blood or urinary ßHCG (exclude pregnancy)
Complete blood count (Evaluate blood loss, search for low platelet count)
Prothrombin time (PT), and the activated partial thromboplastin time
Prolactin, Thyroid Stimulating Hormone (if ovulatory disorder suspected)
Vaginal swab for screening of pelvic infections

Other investigation should be based on the findings of these initial tests and include;

1. Endocrine disorders contribute to abnormal uterine bleeding, tests to determine ovulatory status may be recommended to determine if the woman ovulates during each monthly cycle.
2. Structural abnormalities such as uterine fibroids or polyps and Premalignant and malignant lesion of the endometrium are common causes of AUB. Investigations that will assess the endometrium may be performed to exclude them.
   a. Endometrial biopsy may be performed in women age 45 or older to exclude endometrial cancer or abnormal endometrial growths. In women less than 45 years but at risk for endometrial cancer or infection like tuberculosis should also have a biopsy.
   b. Transvaginal ultrasound can be used to evaluate and measure the uterine lining, it cannot distinguish between polyp and cancer. If these conditions are suspected further testing may be necessary.
   c. Hysteroscopy allow the physician to have a direct view of the inside of the uterus. Tissue samples may be taken.
   d. Dilation and curettage procedure is used to remove endometrial or uterine tissue. It can sometimes be used as a treatment for prolonged or excessive bleeding that is due to hormonal changes and that is unresponsive to other treatments.

Treatment of abnormal uterine bleeding: The treatment of abnormal uterine bleeding is based upon the underlying cause.

- Surgery. In AUB patient with structural abnormality, surgery may be necessary to remove them. Also for those who have completed childbearing and have heavy menstrual bleeding hysterectomy or endometrial ablation may be consider. Myomectomy may be performed for those desiring child bearing.
- Contraceptive pills. Used to treat uterine bleeding that is due to hormonal changes or hormonal irregularities. It is used in women who do not ovulate regularly to establish regular bleeding cycles and prevent excessive growth of the endometrium. In those who do ovulate, it can be used to treat excessive menstrual bleeding. During the perimenopausal period oral contraceptives pills may be used to regulate the menstrual cycle and prevent excessive growth of the endometrium.
- Nonsteroidal anti-inflammatory drug. May be used to reduce blood loss and cramping in ovulatory women.

- Progesterone. May be given to prevent excessive growth of the uterine lining and heavy menstrual bleeding. If no bleeding is seen after progestin treatment, the possibility of pregnancy should be explored.

Conclusion

Menstruation marks the beginning of the process by which the uterus, prepares itself for pregnancy. Each month the uterine endometrium is shed, producing a period and a new lining is grown to replace it. The onset of the first menstruation occurs at puberty, termed menarche and its cessation, termed the menopause. Understanding the complex interplay of the hypothalamic–pituitary-ovarian axis and its feedback loops and the resultant effects on the female reproductive organs provides a foundation for family planning, management of infertility and menstrual abnormalities. Until recently, the terms and terminology used in identifying various abnormalities in menstruation were confusing and often ambiguous. "The PALM-COEIN Classification System" was adopted by the Federation International Gynecology Obstetrics (FIGO) in 2010 to harmonise these terminologies. The treatment of AUB is based on the cause.

References

[1] Lobo RA. The menstrual cycle: In: Mischell DR, Davajan V, Lobo RA (ed.). Infertility, contraception and reproductive endocrinology. Blackwell scientific classification. Boston MA. US. 104-124.

[2] Hallberg L, Hogdahl A, Nilsson L, Rybo G. Menstrual blood loss: a population study. *Acta Obstet Gynecol Scand* 1966;45:320-51.

[3] Baerwald AR, Adams, GP, Pierson, RA. Characterisation of ovarian follicular wave dynamics in women. *Biol Reprod.* 2003; 69:1023-31.

[4] Lui Y, Gold EB, Lasley BL, Johnson WO. Factors affecting menstrual cycle characteristics. *Am J Epidemiol.* 2004; 160(2):131-40.

[5] Arevalo M, Sinai I, Jennings V: A fixed formula to define the fertile window of the menstrual cycle as the basis of a simple method of NFP. *Contraception* 60:357-360, 1999.

[6] Pyper, C, Knight, J, *Glob. libr. Women's med., (ISSN: 1756-2228)* 2008; DOI 10.3843/GLOWM.10384.

[7] Stebbings WSL, Farthing MJG, Anderson E, Puddyfoot JR, Vinson GP, Wood FM. Sex steroid receptor status in colorectal cancer in relation to serum sex and pituitary hormone concentrations and survival. *Gastroenterology* 1987; 92: 1653.

[8] Bernstein et al.: Gastrointestinal symptoms before and during menses in healthy women. *BMC Women's Health* 2014 14:14.

[9] Dajani EZ, Shahwan TG, Dajani NE: Prostaglandins and brain-gut axis. *J Physiol Pharmacol* 2003, 54(Suppl. 4):155-164.

[10] X.A.K Janse de Jonge, C.R.L Boot, J.M. Thom, P.A. Ruell and M.W. Thompson. The influence of menstrual cycle phase on skeletal muscle contractile characteristics in humans. *Journal of physiology* 2001. 530.1, pp. 161-166.

[11] Sato N, Miyake S, Akatsu J AND Kumashiro M. Power spectrum analysis of heart rate variability in healthy young women during the menstrual cycle. *Psychosomatic medicine* 1995.57 pp 331-335.

[12] K. Sembulingam, Prema Sembulingam. *Essentials of medical physiology sixth edition.* pg 480.

[13] Munro MG. Classification of menstrual bleeding disorders. *Rev Endocr Metab Disord* 2012;13:225-234.

[14] Munro MG, Critchley HOD, Broder MS, Fraser IS. FIGO classification system (PALM-COEIN) for causes of abnormal uterine bleeding in nongravid women of reproductive age. *International Journal of Gynecology and Obstetrics* 113 (2011) 3-13.

[15] Wamsteker K, Emanuel MH, de Kruif JH. Transcervical hysteroscopic resection of submucous fibroids for abnormal uterine bleeding: Results regarding the degree of intramural extension. *Obstet Gynecol.* 1993;82(5):736-40.

[16] Mohamed K, Khaled T. Diagnosis and Management of Formerly Called "Dysfunctional Uterine Bleeding" According to PALM-COEIN FIGO Classification and the New Guidelines. *The Journal of Obstetrics and Gynecology of India* (November-December 2014; 64(6):388-393.

In: Amenorrhea
Editor: Oliver Chukwujekwu Ezechi
ISBN: 978-1-63484-778-0

Chapter 3

EVALUATION OF AMENORRHEA

Oliver Chukwujekwu Ezechi
Division of Clinical Sciences, Nigerian Institute of Medical Research,
Yaba Lagos, Nigeria

ABSTRACT

Amenorrhea results from a number of different pathological condition and even physiologic state such as pregnancy and lactation. Systematic step by step evaluations that include patient's medical history, physical examination, and investigations usually identify the underlying cause. Physiologic states like pregnancy and menopause should always be excluded in all cases. The list of pathological causes of amenorrhea is long and includes anatomical or functional anomalies of the genital tract, hormonal disorders, and multifactorial reasons. Basic investigations should include a pregnancy test, assay of serum levels of gonadotropin release hormones, prolactin, thyroid-stimulating hormone, pelvic ultrasound and hysterosalpingography especially in low resource setting were endoscopic investigations are not readily available. Further investigations depend on the outcome of this initial workup. The distinction between primary and secondary amenorrhea, together with the presence, or absence of secondary sexual characteristic development will guide the clinician to possible cause of amenorrhea.

Keywords: amenorrhea, evaluation, diagnois, investigation, medical history

INTRODUCTION

A number of physiologic and pathologic conditions could lead to amenorrhea. Each of these conditions is associated with varying symptomatology and clinical manifestation. It is important to consider a broad range of conditions during evaluation to avoid missing rare or emergent condition. In young females, evaluation should be start if they fail to achieve puberty by 13 years of age, menarche has not occurred five years after initial breast development or by 15 years of age. For women that have achieved menarche, evaluation should also be commenced if there is cessation of previously regular menses for 3 months or previously irregular menses for 6 months [1, 2].

The distinction between primary and secondary amenorrhea is of little importance because there is considerable overlap in aetiology and physical examination. A careful and detailed history and physical examination is what is required as in significant number of patients the diagnosis can be suspected even early in the work up. The anatomic causes of amenorrhea are relatively few, and the majority may be diagnosed by history and physical examination [1].

A systematic step by step evaluations and consideration of the possible causes of amenorrhea by categories is usually helpful in identifying the cause of amenorrhea (Table 1).

Table 1. Common causes of amenorrhea

Physiologic	**Pathologic**	
1. Breastfeeding 2. Contraception 3. Exogenous androgens 4. Menopause 5. Pregnancy	Outflow tract 1. Congenital Complete androgen resistance Imperforate hymen Müllerian agenesis Transverse vaginal septum 2. Acquired Asherman syndrome Cervical stenosis	Primary ovarian insufficiency 1. Congenital Gonadal dysgenesis Turner syndrome 2. Acquired Autoimmune destruction Chemotherapy or radiation Pituitary 1. Autoimmune disease 2. Drugs – Cocaine 3. Cushing syndrome 4. Hyperprolactinaemia 5. Medications e.g., antidepressants, antipsychotics, antihypertensive 6. Sheehan's syndrome
	Hypothalamic 1. Eating disorders 2. Kallmann syndrome 3. Infections e.g., uberculosis 4. Traumatic brain injury 5. Tumour	Other endocrine gland 1. Adrenal disease 2. Constitutional delay 3. Ovarian tumours 4. Polycystic ovarian disease 5. Thyroid

MEDICAL HISTORY

Attending physician should always remember that a thorough medical history is an essential starting point of the evaluation of patients with amenorrhea. It should include information about family medical history, the age of menarche and any underlying systemic disease. Circumstances surrounding pubertal development should be reviewed in details. Age at menarche? Did the patient achieve normal pubertal development? Did the menstrual cycle normalise after few years after menarche? In patients with primary amenorrhea, the presence of developed secondary sexual characteristics is important and demonstrates that sexual steroids are formed and circulating. It is important to determine when the change in menstrual pattern was first noted and how it progressed to the current state. Is it a gradual or sudden occurrence? Any association with pelvic infection, surgery or radiotherapy, child birth or head trauma?

A comprehensive review of all the systems is important as some symptomatology in other system may be a pointer to the cause of amenorrhea. Finally obtaining social and substance use history is important as some social behaviour and habits may cause amenorrhea, e.g., use of cocaine and obsession with dieting and weight loss.

Physical Examination

A detail physical examination after a comprehensive medical history often provides a working diagnosis. This systematic approach to disease diagnosis assists in limiting the number of investigations, reduce time to diagnosis as well as reduce the overall cost of patient management. Physical examination of patients, should be systematic and performed in the following order; general, systemic and genital examination. During the physical examination particular attention should be paid in searching for signs or symptoms of systemic diseases.

Physical examination should be thorough and meticulously performed.

General appearance of the patient may be a pointer to possible aetiology of primary amenorrhea, as with few exceptions physical signs of the cause are so apparent in the diagnosis [1-3].

On breast examination, bilateral galactorrhoea implies the presence of hyperprolactinemia. This should prompt examination of the visual field if not done already. Finding of bitemporal hemianopia may be indicative of a tumour in the pituitary gland. However, it is important to note that the absence of galactorrhoea does not exclude hyperprolactinaemia.

Examination of genital should start with the observation of the hair pattern, confirmation of the presence or absence of the hymen and vaginal canal. This is followed by digital examination to verify the anatomic integrity of the uterus and the absence of palpable masses at the adnexa. In patients that are vago intact, per rectum bimanual evaluation will provide the same information. Always use the opportunity to screening for cervical and other genital cancer [4, 5].

Investigation

To the inexperience because of the long list of causes of amenorrhea, deciphering the cause in a particular patient seems daunting. Fortunately, evaluation of most patients is straightforward. Flexibility rather than sticking to a very rigid schema is important to timely diagnosis. How to proceed with the investigation should depend mainly on the history and physical examination findings. The basic test includes pregnancy test and determination of serum luteinizing hormone, follicle-stimulating hormone, prolactin, and thyroid-stimulating hormone levels (Table 2). If medical history and or physical examination points to a hyperandrogenic state, patient should be evaluated for increased androgens using serum free and total testosterone and dehydroepiandrosterone sulfate concentrations. Serum estradiol should be measured if physical examination shows evidence of poor or no breast development. Short statured patients should be evaluated for Turner syndrome by performing a karyotype analysis [1-6]. In suspected chronic medical condition as a cause, a complete blood count and comprehensive metabolic panel are helpful.

Table 2. Common investigation in the evaluation of amenorrhea

β HCG	**Pregnancy**
Follicle stimulating Hormone	Hypogonadotropic vs Hypergonadotropic hypogonadism
Oestradiol	
Prolactin	Hyperprolactinaemi
Thyroid stimulating hormone	Thyroid disease (hypothyroidism)
Secondary Investigations	
Testosterone	Polycystic ovarian diseases and exclude ovarian tumour
Dehydroepiandrosterone sulfate	Exclude adrenal tumour
17 hydroxy progesterone	Late onset congenital adrenal hyperplasia
2 hours glucose tolerance test	Polycystic ovarian diseases
Autoimmune testing	Premature ovarian failure
Karotype	Turners syndrome, Premature ovarian syndrome
Radiologic examination	
HSG	Müllerian anomaly and Ashermans syndrome
Sonography	Polycystic ovarian diseases, presence of uterus
Magnetic Image Resonance	Müllerian anomaly or hypothalamic pituitary disease

Pelvic ultrasonography can help confirm the presence or absence of a uterus, and can identify structural abnormalities of reproductive tract organs. In low income setting, a hysterosalpingography and intravenous urography will assist in identifying congenital structural abnormalities. MRI is useful in exclude prolactinoma and other pituitary tumours as the cause of amenorrhea.

Progesterone challenge test is helpful in confirming functional anatomy and adequate oestrogenization. However some experts defer this testing because its correlation with estrogen status is relatively unreliable [2-4].

CONCLUSION

The distinction between primary and secondary amenorrhea is of little importance because there is considerable overlap in aetiology and physical examination. A careful and detailed history and physical examination is what is required as in significant number of patients the diagnosis can be suspected even early in the work up. Flexibility rather than sticking to a very rigid schema is important to timely diagnosis. Investigation requested should depend mainly on the history and physical examination findings. The basic test in the investigation of a patient with amenorrhea should include pregnancy test in women of reproductive age, serum luteinizing hormone, follicle-stimulating hormone, prolactin, and thyroid-stimulating hormone levels. Other secondary and tertiary investigation should depend on the finding from these basic tests.

REFERENCES

[1] Klein DA, Poth MA. Amenorrhea: an approach to diagnosis and management. *Am Fam Physician* 2013; 87(11), 781-8.

[2] Practice Committee of American Society for Reproductive Medicine. Current evaluation of amenorrhea. *Fertil Steril.* 2008;90(5): S219-S225.

[3] American College of Obstetricians and Gynecologists. *Amenorrhea (ACOG Technical Bulletin 128).* Washington, D.C.: ACOG, 1989.

[4] Speroff L, Fritz MA. Amenorrhea. In: *Clinical gynecologic endocrinology and infertility.* 7th ed. Philadelphia, Pa.: Lippincott Williams and Wilkins, 2005;401-64.

[5] Bachmann G, Kemmann E. Prevalence of oligomenorrhea and amenorrhea in a college population. *Am J Obstet Gynecol* 1982; 144: 98-102.

[6] Master-Hunter T, Heiman DL. Amenorrhea: evaluation and treatment. *Am Fam Physician* 2006;73:1374-82, 1387.

In: Amenorrhea
Editor: Oliver Chukwujekwu Ezechi
ISBN: 978-1-63484-778-0

Chapter 4

PHARMACOTHERAPY OF AMENORRHEA

Getnet Yimer Ali[1], Alemayehu Toma[2] and Yifru Berhan[3]
[1]Department of Pharmacology, College of Health Sciences,
School of Medicine, Addis Ababa University, Addis Ababa, Ethiopia
[2]Department of Pharmacology, School of Medicine, College of Medicine and Health Sciences, Hawassa University, Hawassa, Ethiopia
[3]Obstetrics and Gynaecology, School of Medicine,
College of Medicine and Health Sciences,
Hawassa University, Hawassa, Ethiopia

ABSTRACT

The pharmacological therapy of amenorrhea is cause and fertility need specific. Identifying the underlying cause of amenorrhea should be priority to make the treatment modality specific and curative. Pharmacological treatment of amenorrhea is only effective after the underlying cause of amenorrhea is treated. For those women who are not desirous of childbearing reassurance alone may suffice, after confirming that the underlying cause of amenorrhea has no other health risk. In those that are desirous of child bearing different management modiatlies including pharmacotherapy are essential.

Keywords: pharmacotherapy, pharmacology, drugs, amenorrhea

INTRODUCTION

The pharmacological therapy of amenorrhea is cause and fertility need specific. For those women who do not plan to have a biological child and if the underlying cause of amenorrhea has no other health risk, pharmacological treatment may not be important; reassuring alone may suffice. In case of amenorrhea associated with organic lesion, treatment should be directed to the underlying pathology. This is because; amenorrhea by itself is not a disease; it is usually a symptom of an underlying anatomic, hormonal or neural disorder. Thus, the treatment of amenorrhea has to be tailored according to the etiology. However, it should be noted that there are conditions where there may not be any identifiable organic lesion associated with amenorrhea, but can have a deleterious effect to the victim. The good examples are athletic amenorrhea and premature ovarian failure, in which deficiency of estrogen and leptin oftentimes results in bone loss, potentially leading to osteoporosis.

On the other hand, if the patient becomes amenorrheic because she is taking hormone replacement or oral contraceptives, that is not, in itself, harmful. Apart from this scenario and pregnancy, however, the majorities of pathological causes of amenorrhea bring about serious health consequences. Depending on the cause, the most common complications include: lack of secondary sexual characteristics, loss of feminine gender identification, central nervous system neoplasia, other endocrinopathies, osteoporosis, cardiovascular disease, and psychiatric disorders. Treatment therefore should not be unduly delayed. Most treatments are aimed at restoring regular menses or physiologic hormone replacement, even if the underlying etiology has not been corrected.

For those patients who wish to conceive, clearly the first goal of treatment would be to initiate ovulation induction. In some cases, such as hyperprolactinemia, medical or surgical correction of the underlying problem will correct the menstrual cycle. For women with the polycyctic ovarian syndrome (PCOS), some may need only ovulation induction with medications such as clomiphene citrate, but others may require more intensive assisted reproduction such as *in vitro* fertilization (IVF). Pregnancy is difficult, but not impossible in women with premature ovarian failure too.

Treatment options for amenorrhea may include dietary modifications (increase in fat and carbohydrate intake in order to stimulate estrogen production), psychotherapy for eating disorders, applying stress reduction techniques, hormonal analogue supplementation, surgical excision of outflow tract obstruction or hormone producing adenomas. As usual, identifying the underlying cause of amenorrhea is given priority to make the treatment modality specific and curative.

Likewise, the pharmacological treatment of amenorrhea will be effective if the underlying cause is clearly identified.

DRUG TREATMENT

Selective Serotonin Reuptake Inhibitors

Hypothalamus, as a source of GnRh, function is influenced by multiple factors affecting the function of the brain cortex (anorexia nervosa, excessive exercise or physical stress, psychosocial stress, malnutrition, chronic illness, drugs etc.).

Studies have provided that the administration of a selective serotonin reuptake inhibitors (SSRI) might correct abnormalities of Functional Hypothalamic Amenorrhea (FHA), particularly stress-related. Their mechanism involves the repair of the P13K signaling pathway, which in turn facilitates the integration of metabolic and neural signals to regulate gonadotropin releasing hormone (GnRH). In other words, SSRIs regulate the neuronal activity and expression of neuropeptide systems and promote GnRH release. SSRI therapy is an advantage for a possible hormonal regulation of hypothalamic amenorrhea.

Metreleptin (r-metHuLeptin) is a prototype SSRI for treatment of stress related hypothalamic amenorrhea. R-metHuLeptin has also been tested as a treatment for estrogen deficiency due to low gonadotropins and low concentrations of thyroid hormone and IGF-1.

The result has shown its effectiveness in restoring defects in the hypothalamic-pituitary-gonadal axis and improving reproductive performance, thyroid and IGF hormones production and bone formation, with the cumulative effect of menstrual regularity and restoring fertility. However, it was not effective in restoring of cortisol and adrenocoticotropin production and bone resorption.

Metformin

Metformin decreases resistance to the hormone insulin, as well as levels of prolactin, testosterone, and lutenizing hormone (LH). Metformin also decreases the LH/FSH ratio.

The regulation of these hormones implicates the correction of secondary amenorrhea.

Clinical trials on patients with PCOS demonstrated that the majority of patients in the Metformin group had resumed regular menses because of accompanying reduction in insulin and testosterone level.

GnRH Analogues

For women with hypothalamic amenorrhea who desire pregnancy, ovulation induction with pulsatile GnRH or injectable gonadotropins is the treatment of choice. A retrospective analysis of 30 women receiving gonadotropin therapy and 41 receiving pulsatile GnRH therapy showed ovulatory rates of 93% to 97%, respectively. GnRH therapy was associated with a lower rate of multiple gestations than gonadotropin therapy. Estrogen-deficient women with hypothalamic amenorrhea often have a poor response to ovulation induction with clomiphene citrate. In one study involving eight women, priming with estrogen plus progestin appeared to improve the ovulation rate after the administration of clomiphene, although this approach requires further study. The pattern of hypogonadotropic hypogonadism is not fixed in such patients, and responses may vary, depending on weight and estrogen status. Limited data indicate that leptin and opioid antagonists may restore ovulation in women with hypothalamic amenorrhea.

Dopamine Agonists

Dopamine agonists are the preferred treatment for most patients with hyperprolactinemic disorders; these agents are extremely effective in lowering serum prolactin levels, eliminating galactorrhea, restoring regular menses and decreasing tumor size. The two most commonly prescribed drugs in the treatment of hyperprolactinemia are bromocriptine and cabergoline. They are dopamine receptor agonists and share many characteristics and adverse effects, such as headache, nausea and vomiting, though the frequency and severity of adverse effects appear to be less in cabergoline compared to bromocriptine group. Studies demonstrated that cabergoline was significantly better than bromocriptine in decreasing the risks of persistent hyperprolactinemia, amenorrhea/oligomenorrhea and galactorrhea. Frequency of dosing may also affect treatment decisions as cabergoline is dosed twice weekly, whereas bromocriptine is given daily. However, cabergoline costs at least twice as much as bromocriptine and was not found to be superior in other outcomes. Though both drugs have been found to be safe in pregnancy, the number of reports studying bromocriptine in pregnancy far exceeds that of cabergoline in pregnancy.

A large body of moderate quality evidence from observational studies supports the use of dopamine agonists to normalize prolactin levels and resolve the symptoms related to mass effect and elevated prolactin levels. The large treatment effect of dopamine agonists, the potential dose response effect, biological plausibility, temporality between treatment and effect, consistency across studies, settings and methods, and coherence (consistency across agents within the same class), strongly support the effectiveness of these treatment agents in reducing prolactin levels and improving symptoms.

Leptin Analogue

Circulating leptin levels reflect the amount of energy stores in fat as well as acute changes in energy intake. Hypoleptinemia, signaling a state of energy deficiency, may mediate the changes in the neuroendocrine axes observed in hypothalamic amenorrhea. Inadequate nutrition delays or prevents the onset of puberty. Leptin acts as a permissive signal to activate the reproductive axis. Leptin accelerates GnRH – pulsatility in arcute hypothalamic neurons regulating the release of ganadotropin. It was indicated that acutely depriving of energy by caloric restriction resulted in a relative leptin deficiency and neuroendocrine abnormalities affecting the gonadal and thyroid axes, and these abnormalities were prevented with recombinant methionyl human leptin (metreleptin) replacement.

Exogenous leptin may be relatively more effective in subjects in whom endogenous leptin production has first been reduced by dieting. Women with hypothalamic amenorrhea are chronically energy deficient, have low leptin levels and loss of diurnal leptin variation. Metreleptin administration normalized leptin levels in women with hypothalamic amenorrhea and found that metreleptin treatment resulted in ovulatory menses and significant increases in levels of luteinizing hormone (LH), estradiol, insulin-like growth factor-1 (IGF1), thyroid hormones, and bone formation markers.

REFERENCES

Ahmed J., Isam H., Zena S. (2008). Comparison of the effects of cabergoline and bromocriptine in women with hyperprolactinemic amenorrhea. *MEFSJ,* 13: 33-38.

Bacopoulou F., Creatsas G., Chrousos G., Papanikolaou N., Deligeoroglou E. (2014). Primary amenorrhea in adolescent girls: normal coitus or not? Always take a look in the physician's office. *BMC Women's Health*, 14:23.

Bahceci M., Sismanoglu A., Ulug U. (2010). Comparison of cabergoline and bromocriptine in patients with asymptomatic incidental hyperprolactinemia undergoing ICSI-ET. *Gynecol. Endocrinol.*, 26:505–508.

De Luis D. A., Becerra A., Lahera M., Botella J. I., Valero M. A., Varela C. (2000). A randomized coss-over study comparing cabergoline and quinagolide in the treatment of hyperprolactinemic patients. *J. Endocrinol. Invest.,* 23: 428-434.

Fourman, L. T. and P. K. Fazeli (2015). "Neuroendocrine causes of amenorrhea--an update." J. Clin. Endocrinol. Metab., 100: 812-824.

Ghaffari, F., F. Keikha, et al. (2015). "A rare case of primary amenorrhea with two etiologies, hypothalamic amenorrhea, transverse vaginal septum, and no hematocolpos." Case Rep. Obstet. Gynecol., 9, 89-123.

Gruen, P. H., Sachar, E. J., Altman, N., et al. (1978). Neuroleptic drugs. *Endocrinology and Metabolism Clinics of North America*, 17, 213-223.

Gruender, G.,Wetzel, H., Schloesser, R., et al. (1999) Relation of plasma prolactin to clinical response in schizophrenic patients. *Archives of General Psychiatry*, 35, 1222-1227.

Haddad, P. and Wieck, A. (2000). Neuroendocrine response to antipsychotics: effects of drug type and gender. *Biological Psychiatry*, 45, 89^97.

Halbreich, U., Rojansky, N., Palter, S., et al. (1995); Antipsychotic-induced hyperprolactinaemia: a series of illustrative case reports. *Journal of Psychopharmacology*, 15, 293-295.

Jabeen, S. and M. Raees (2015). "Primary amenorrhea with bilateral endometriotic cysts." *J. Coll. Physicians Surg. Pak.,* 25: 372-373.

Kinon, B. and Gilmore, J. (2001); Risperidone and associated amenorrhea: a report of 5 cases. *Journal of Clinical Psychiatry*, 60, 315-317.

Kleinberg, D. L., Davis, J. M., De Coster, R., et al. (1999) Prevalence of hyperprolactinemia in a large cohort of schizophrenic patients treated with conventional antipsychotic drugs or risperidone. *Archives of Women's Mental Health,* 3 (suppl. 2), S185.

Klibanski, A. and Greenspan, S. L. (1986); Prolactin levels and adverse effects in patients treated with risperidone. *Journal of Clinical Psychopharmacology,* 19, 57-61.

Kouyate, R. A., S. Ahmed, et al. (2015). "Transition from the Lactational Amenorrhea Method to other modern family planning methods in rural Bangladesh: barrier analysis and implications for behavior change communication program intervention design." *Eval. Program Plann.*, 50: 10-17.

Marsh, C. A. and F. W. Grimstad (2014). "Primary amenorrhea: diagnosis and management." *Obstet. Gynecol. Surv.,* 69(10): 603-612.

Mohebbi-Kian, E., S. Mohammad-Alizadeh-Charandabi, et al. (2014). "Efficacy of fennel and combined oral contraceptive on depot medroxyprogesterone acetate-induced amenorrhea: a randomized placebo-controlled trial." *Contraception,* 90(4): 440-446.

Motazedian S., Babakhani L., Fereshtehnejad S. M., Mojtahedi K. (2010). A comparison of bromocriptine and cabergoline on fertility outcome of hyperprolactinemic infertile women undergoing intrauterine insemination. *Indian J. Med. Res.,* 131: 670–674.

Valassi E., Klibanski A., Biller B. (2010). Clinical Review#: Potential cardiac valve effects of dopamine agonists in hyperprolactinemia. *J. Clin. Endocrinol. Metab.*, 95: 1025–1033.

Verhelst J., Abs R. (2003). Hyperprolactinemia: pathophysiology and management. *Treatments in Endocrinology*, 2003; 2: 23-32.

Wang T., Mullan J., et al. (2012). Treatment of hyperprolactinemia: asystematic review and meta-analysis. *BMC Systematic Reviews*, 1:33.

SECTION II: PRIMARY AMENORRHEA

In: Amenorrhea
Editor: Oliver Chukwujekwu Ezechi
ISBN: 978-1-63484-778-0

Chapter 5

MANAGEMENT OF AMENORRHEA IN ADOLESCENTS

Titilola Abike Gbajabiamila, Agatha Eileen Wapmuk and Oliver Chukwujekwu Ezechi
Division of Clinical Sciences,
Nigerian Institute of Medical Research,
Yaba, Lagos, Nigeria

ABSTRACT

Menstrual disorders such as amenorrhea are particularly common in adolescent girls and often the source of anxiety for the patients and the families. Although menstrual irregularities may be normal during the early post menarchal years, complete absence or cessation of menses, requires careful evaluation and management. Amenorrhea except that occurring before puberty, during pregnancy or early lactation, and after menopause is pathologic. Amenorrhea in an adolescent could be primary or secondary and may be caused by anatomic abnormalities; hypothalamic, pituitary, or other endocrine dysfunction; ovarian failure; or genetic defects. However, the most common causes are hypothalamic amenorrhea, polycystic ovarian disease, hyperprolactinemia, and ovarian failure. A detailed review of medical history and careful clinical examination of the young girl is absolutely essential. A physician should be guided towards making diagnosis of the cause of amenorrhea by identifying from the history the type of amenorrhea (primary and secondary), together with presence or absence of secondary sexual characteristic. Basic laboratory investigation should include gonadotropin release hormones, and prolactin measurements; while in the presence of acne or hirsutism, androgen levels should also be measured. Treatment should be focused at restoration of ovulatory cycle and prevention of short- and long-term consequences of oestrogen deficiency.

Keywords: adolescence, puberty, menarche, amenorrhea, menstrual cycle

INTRODUCTION

Adolescence is a transitional stage, characterized by major mental and physical changes. Puberty and menarche in girls is unquestionably the most significant body change occurring during this period. The age of menarche continue to decline since the last century and in high income countries, it usually occurs between the ages of 12 and 13 years. Similar trend have also been noticed in low and middle income countries as standard of living improved over the years [1].

The length of the normal menstrual cycle is highly variable. Normal menstrual cycles are characterized by a cycle length of 28 days, a duration of flow of 4.5 days, and a blood loss of less than 80 mL.

Menstrual cycles are abnormal if they are longer than 8 days in duration or if more than 80 mL of blood loss occurs, especially in the early years after menarche. Abnormal or irregular menstrual patterns are common in the early adolescent period and the variability in cycle length is greater compared to variability during adulthood [1, 2]. As the menstrual cycle is the result of a complex interaction between the various organs, abnormality at any level may interfere with ovulation and the menstruation. Thus amenorrhea except that occurring before puberty, during pregnancy or early lactation is pathologic.

The most common aetiology of amenorrhea in adolescent is dysfunction of the hypothalamic-pituitary-ovarian axis. A careful history, a detailed examination and appropriate investigations are necessary to diagnose these adolescents properly. The management depends on the aetiologies of the problems and involves surgical correction, hormone replacement and other appropriate medical therapies accordingly [1-4].

PUBERTY

The mechanism for initiating puberty in late childhood is incompletely understood. What is known is that for some reason, the hypothalamus becomes less sensitive to circulating gonadal hormones. The GnRH pulses increase in amplitude and frequency and are followed by pulses of LH and FSH. In response to rising LH and FSH levels, the ovary produces estrogen, which initiates sexual maturation, heralded by the development of breast (thelarche). There is a normal progression of pubertal development in girls. In girls, menarche usually occurs during late stage of breast development and usually lags behind thelarche by 2-3 years. It takes about 5 years after menarche for the establishment of regular menstrual cycles [2, 3]. The interval between the first menstrual and second period can be quite long, but subsequent cycles usually vary from 21 to 45 days, with very few cycles occurring outside of this range. In the years after menarche, the cycles are typically anovulatory accounting for the wide variation in the length of the cycle during this phase of development. Once the hypothalamo-pituitary-ovarian axis matures, the pattern of menstrual cycle normalises as the cycle becomes increasingly ovulatory [2-4].

PATHOGENESIS

Menstrual cycle is an orderly progression of coordinated hormonal events in the female body that stimulates growth of a follicle to release an egg and prepare a site for implantation if fertilization should occur [4, 5]. Menstruation occurs when an egg released by the ovary remains unfertilized; subsequently, the soggy decidua of the endometrium sloughed in a flow of menses in preparation for another cycle [6, 7].

Hypothalamus, pituitary and ovaries form a functional endocrine axis, known as HPO axis with hormonal regulations and feedback loops [7]. The normal function of this endocrine axis is required for Menarche and sustained menstrual cycles. Any disruption in this axis may result in amenorrhea. Defining the level of primary dysfunction is critical in determining the pathophysiology of amenorrhea.

At birth, female infants have a predetermined number of primordial follicles that are arrested during meiosis 1 at the diplotene stage of prophase until stimulation at puberty. Until puberty, the hypothalamus is in a dormant state. At about age 8 years, gonadotropin-releasing hormone (GnRH) is synthesized in the hypothalamus and released [3]. The adrenal cortex begins to produce dehydroepiandrostenedione to initiate the start of adrenarche [6].

The orderly progression of puberty begins with breast budding, accelerated growth, and menses. Pubarche, which is independent from GnRH function, typically occurs between breast budding and accelerated growth but may occur anywhere along the puberty timeline.

Menarche and sustained menstrual cycles requires normal function of the endocrine axis comprising the hypothalamus, pituitary, and ovaries [1, 4].

CAUSES OF AMENORRHEA

Amenorrhea in adolescents can be caused by anatomic abnormalities; hypothalamic, pituitary, or other endocrine dysfunction; ovarian failure; or genetic defects (Table 1).

Anatomic Defects of the Outflow Tract

A patent vaginal tract and a functional uterus are needed for normal menstrual flow to occur. Genital tract abnormalities account for about 20% of all cases of primary amenorrhea [6]. Cyclic pelvic pain is common in girls with disorders of the reproductive tract involving outflow obstruction. Imperforate hymen causes an outflow obstruction. These patients can have blood in the vagina that collects and can result in a perirectal mass. Transverse vaginal septum is another cause of out flow tract obstruction and can be found anywhere along the vagina between the hymenal ring and uterine cervix [4, 6].

Mayer-Rokitansky-Kuster-Hauser (MRKH) syndrome is another cause of genital tract abnormality presenting as primary amenorrhea. In MRKH there is vaginal agenesis caused by agenesis or partial agenesis of the müllerian duct system [8]. It is characterized by congenital aplasia of the uterus and upper two thirds of the vagina in women with developed secondary sexual characteristics and a normal 46, XX karyotype [8]. The first sign is primary amenorrhea. It affects 1 of 4500 women and can be associated with renal, vertebral, auditory and cardiac defects [8-11].

Table 1. Common causes of amenorrhea in adolescents

Group Classification	Specific Conditions
Anatomic defects of the outflow tract	• Müllerian agenesis • Complete androgen resistance • Imperforate hymen • Transverse vaginal septum • Cervical agenesis—isolated • Vaginal agenesis—isolated • Congenital endometrial hypoplasia or aplasia
Primary hypogonadism	• Gonadal dysgenesis • Premature ovarian failure, • FSH or LH receptor mutations • Enzymatic deficiencies
Hypothalamic causes	• Functional hypothalamic amenorrhea. • Isolated gonadotropin deficiency • Kallmann syndrome • Idiopathic hypogonadotropic hypogonadism • Infection (tuberculosis,sarcoidosis) • Brain tumors • Chronic systemic illness
Pituitary causes	• Prolactinomas • Craniopharyngioma • Empty sella syndrome • Pituitary necrosis • Panhypopituitarism

Pituitary Amenorrhea

A deficiency in gonadotropins may result from GnRH receptor gene mutations, although such mutations are rare. Mutations in the FSH beta gene have also been associated with amenorrhea; women with these mutations have low FSH and estradiol levels and high LH levels.

Primary amenorrhea caused by hyperprolactinemia is a rare condition characterized by the onset of thelarche and pubarche at appropriate ages but arrest of pubertal development before menarche [12-18]. Hyperprolactinemia is associated with suppression of the GnRH from the hypothalamus and subsequent inhibition of LH and FSH, suppressed gonadal function and galactorrhea [19, 20]. Prolactinomas are more commonly noted in secondary amenorrhea [23].

Pituitary tumours may suppress gonadotropin secretion, such as in Cushing disease or hypothalamic tumours, craniopharyngioma, or germinoma [20, 21]. Brain injury or cranial irradiation may also result in amenorrhea.

Gonadal dysgenesis is characterized by the congenital loss or underdevelopment of germ cells within the gonad during organogenesis [22]. The gonads usually contain only fibrous tissue and are called streak gonads. In females, the most common form of gonadal dysgenesis is Turner syndrome (45, X), in which gonadotropin levels, especially the FSH levels, are high during early childhood and after age 9-10 years. Depletion of ovarian follicles causes amenorrhea. Premature ovarian failure should be investigated if suspected. The fragile X permutation accounts for approximately 6% of cases of overt POF [23]). Autoimmune oophoritis occurs in 3-4% of POF cases.

Amenorrhea is also seen in pure 46, XX gonadal dysgenesis and in 46, XY gonadal dysgenesis. These women have significantly elevated FSH levels due to the absence of ovarian follicles and reduction in negative feedback on FSH from estradiol and inhibin A and B [6]. Polycystic ovarian syndrome (PCOS) usually presents as secondary amenorrhea, but in some cases may present as primary amenorrhea [23-25].

Hypothalamic Amenorrhea

Hypothalamic amenorrhea which is the most prevalent cause of amenorrhea in the adolescent age group. It occurs as a result in decreased or inhibited GnRH secretion, which affects the pulsatile release of pituitary gonadotropins, LH and FSH, causing anovulation. Functional hypothalamic amenorrhea is a common cause of amenorrhea [10]. It is characterized by abnormal hypothalamic GnRH secretion, decreased gonadotropin pulsations, low or normal LH concentrations, absent LH surges, abnormal follicular development, and low serum estradiol. It is important to note that the Serum FSH concentrations are usually in the normal range, with high FSH-to-LH ratio [10].

Functional hypothalamic amenorrhea can be caused by eating disorders, exercise, or high levels of prolonged physical or mental stress. This can also include major psychiatric disorders such as depression. Hypothyroidism, hyperthyroidism, sarcoidosis, galactosemia or any severe chronic medical condition may result in amenorrhea [10].

Idiopathic hypogonadotropic hypogonadism leads to low gonadotropin (FSH/LH) levels [11]. When this occurs with anosmia, it is diagnosed as Kallmann syndrome, the signs of which include midline facial defects, renal agenesis, and neurologic deficiencies [12]. Kallmann syndrome results from a failure of GnRH cells to migrate to the forebrain, a phenomenon associated with mutations in the genes KAL1, FGFR1, FGF8, PROKR2, and PROK2 [11, 14].

Evidence suggests a negative correlation between body fat levels and menstrual abnormalities. A critical body fat level must be present for the reproductive system to function normally. In some female athletes, the synergistic effects of excessive exercise and disordered eating cause severe suppression of GnRH, leading to low estradiol levels [15, 16].

Anorexia nervosa is a serious psychiatric disease with severe medical complications including primary amenorrhea, osteopenia, and osteoporosis [19]. Though amenorrhea is currently being used as a Diagnostic Criterion for Anorexia Nervosa [17]. Some researchers have said that based on existing evidence it may be removed as a diagnostic criterion.

Functional causes of amenorrhea include severe chronic disease, rapid weight loss, malnutrition, depression or other psychiatric disorders, recreational drug abuse, and psychotropic drug use [1].

Receptor and Enzyme Defects

Congenital adrenal hyperplasia as a result of 17 alpha-hydroxylase deficiency (CYP17) causes an excess of deoxycortisone to be produced and deficiency of cortisol and adrenal and gonadal sex steroids [26]. Patients with this disorder who experience primary amenorrhea can be either genotypic males (XY) or females (XX) [26].

Complete androgen insensitivity syndrome is caused by a defective androgen receptor. Although patients with this syndrome have a 46, XY karyotype and produce testicularly derived testosterone, the testosterone cannot activate cellular transcription; therefore, the patient has female external genitalia. In most cases the disorder is X-linked. The testes, located internally and sometimes in the labia or inguinal area, also produce müllerian-inhibiting hormone, so all müllerian-derived structures (i.e., the fallopian tubes, uterus, upper third of the vagina) are absent [27].

MANAGEMENT

The assessment of an adolescent amenorrhea requires a sensitive age approach in which the psychosocial age as well as the emotional maturity is considered rather than the chronological maturity. A thorough systematic evaluation including a detailed history, physical examination, and laboratory assessment of selected serum hormone levels is usually done to identify the underlying cause. Management should focus on the restoration of ovulatory cycles and the prevention of short- and long-term consequences of hormonal imbalance.

Medical History: A detailed history will help in narrowing down your differential diagnosis as to what the aetiology of the amenorrhea is. Enquiries should involve reviewing the history of childhood growth and development, obtaining age at thelarche and menarche, and family history to determine age at menarche of mother and female siblings. Duration and flow of menses, cycle days and date of last menstrual period should be obtained. Try eliciting history of a chronic illness such as HIV, sickle cell disease, thalasaemia, diabetes mellitus[i], epilepsy, chronic kidney disease and malignancy. History of trauma, surgery and psychosocial issues should be explored. It is also essential to obtain information on; psychiatric illness, medication, physical activity and sports, sexual behaviour and history.

Physical Examination

The adolescent should be engaged in a discussion to assess her emotional maturity and establish a relationship before commencing the physical examination. The physician should share age-appropriate information about the condition with the adolescent as well as respond to questions by the patient. First assess degree of sexual development, nutritional status and evidence for chronic disease, cachexia or obesity. Specifically look out for the following signs;

- Sweaty palms, tachycardia, hypertension, nervousness which are suggestive of hyperthyroidism
- Short stature, webbed neck, low-set hairline and/or ears, pubertal delay, cubitus valgus, nail hypoplasia, short fourth metacarpal, high-arched palate, chronic otitis media and cardiac abnormalities, which are the stigmata of turners syndrome.
- Hirsutism, hair loss, and acne which are evidence of androgen excess
- Thin, parchment-like skin, wide purplish striae, and evidence of easy bruising as in Cushing syndrome.
- Warm and moist skin radiating excessive heat of hyperthyroidism
- Presence of axillary and pubic hair which are evidence of adrenal and ovarian androgen secretion.
- Adolescents who have a combination of autoimmune premature ovarian failure and autoimmune primary adrenal insufficiency are also markedly androgen deficient and have scant axillary and pubic hair.

Assess for the state of breast development. Underdeveloped breasts with sparse pubic hair are seen in cases of delayed puberty while undeveloped breasts with normal growth of pubic hair are seen in cases of gonadal dysgenesis (eg, Turner syndrome). Also examine the breast for the presence of galactorrhea. A thorough examination of the external genitalia or pelvic examination is required as this may detect ambiguous genitalia, absence or abnormalities of cervix or uterus, presence of transverse vaginal septum, imperforate hymen, reddened or thin vaginal mucosa. Observe and measure the size and length of the clitoris. A clitoral index greater than 100 mm^2 is evidence of virilization. During pelvic examination, ovarian enlargement may be found especially in cases of autoimmune oophoritis or 17-hydroxylase deficiency. Ovarian enlargement is also commonly associated with Polycystic ovarian syndrome [1, 3, 5].

Laboratory Investigations

These are carried out to confirm suspected diagnosis from history and physical examination. Differential diagnosis generated while taking history and physical examinations should guide the choice of investigations. The basic investigations to confirm diagnosis in adolescent with amenorrhea are listed in Table 2.

Treatment

Amenorrhea is a treatable condition; however this depends on some factors which are associated with the aetiology of amenorrhea in adolescents and the desires of the patient. Treatment should be directed at correcting the underlying pathology. In the case of outflow tract abnormalities (e.g., imperforate hymen), surgery may be indicated. In other cases, correcting the underlying pathology should restore normal ovarian endocrine function and prevent short and long term consequences of hormonal imbalance, e.g the development of osteoporosis. The factors listed in table 3 should be considered when treating a patient with amenorrhea [2, 4, 5].

Table 2. Investigation of adolescent with amenorrhea

Type of investigation
Pregnancy test
Complete blood count with diff
Erythrocyte Sedimentation rate
Thyroid function tests
Prolactin
Determination of serum gonadotropins (serum FSH and LH determination)
Progesterone challenge test
Karyotype testing
Bone age film of wrist
Free and total testosterone; dehydroepiandrosterone sulphate (DHEA-S)
Fasting glucose and insulin
Pelvic/abdominal CT Scan or MRI
Magnetic resonance imaging of head or sella

Table 3. Consideration in treating adolescent amenorrhea

Age of the adolescent
Overall health status
Medical history of the adolescent
Extent of the condition
Cause of the condition
Adolescent's tolerance for specific medications, procedures or therapies
Adolescent's opinion or preference

Conclusion

Although menstrual irregularities may be normal during the early post menarchal years, complete absence or cessation of menses, requires careful evaluation and management. The most common causes of adolescent amenorrhea are hypothalamic amenorrhea, polycystic ovarian disease, hyperprolactinemia, and ovarian failure. An attending physician should be guided towards making a diagnosis of the cause of amenorrhea by identifying from the patient's history the type of amenorrhea, together with presence or absence of secondary sexual characteristic. Basic laboratory investigation should include gonadotropin release hormones and prolactin measurements; while in the presence of acne or hirsutism, androgen levels should also be measured. Treatment should be focused at restoration of ovulatory cycle and prevent short- and long-term consequences of oestrogen deficiency.

REFERENCES

[1] Pletcher J. R., Slap G. B. Menstrual disorders: amenorrhea. *Pediatric Clinics of North America,* 1999; 46(3):505-18.

[2] Golden N. H., Carlson J. L. The pathophysiology of amenorrhea in the adolescent. *Annals of the New York Academy of Sciences,* 2008; 1135 (1):163-78.

[3] Deligeoroglou E., Athanasopoulos N., Tsimaris P., Dimopoulos K. D., Vrachnis N., Creatsas G. Evaluation and management of adolescent amenorrhea. *Annals of the New York Academy of Sciences,* 2010; 1205 (1):23-32.

[4] Slap G. B. Menstrual disorders in adolescence. *Best Practice and Research Clinical Obstetrics and Gynaecology,* 2003; 17(1):75-92.

[5] Laroche E., Bricaire L., Christin-Maitre S. [Diagnosis and management of amenorrhea in adolescent girls]. *Archives de pediatrie: organe officiel de la Societe francaise de pediatrie,* 2013; 20(7):817-22.

[6] Rachmiel M., Kives S., Atenafu E., Hamilton J. Primary amenorrhea as a manifestation of polycystic ovarian syndrome in adolescents: a unique subgroup? *Archives of pediatrics and adolescent medicine,* 2008; 162 (6):521-5.

[7] Popat V. B., Prodanov T., Calis K. A., Nelson L. M. The Menstrual Cycle. *Annals of the New York Academy of Sciences*, 2008; 1135 (1): 43-51.

[8] Popat V. B., Prodanov T., Calis K. A., Nelson L. M. The Menstrual Cycle. *Annals of the New York Academy of Sciences*, 2008; 1135 (1): 43-51.

[9] Glueck C. J., Wang P. Age of Menarche and Oligomenorrhea in Adolescence: Cardiometabolic Ramifications in Adulthood. *The Journal of pediatrics,* 2015.

[10] Gordon C. M. Functional hypothalamic amenorrhea. *New England Journal of Medicine*, 2010; 363(4):365-71.

[11] Welt C. K., Barbieri R. Etiology, diagnosis and treatment of secondary amenorrhea. Last literature review version. 2011; 20.

[12] MacColl G., Quinton R., Bouloux P. M. GnRH neuronal development: insights into hypogonadotrophic hypogonadism. *Trends in Endocrinology and Metabolism,* 2002; 13(3):112-8.

[13] Schwanzel-Fukuda M., Bick D., Pfaff D. W. Luteinizing hormone-releasing hormone (LHRH)-expressing cells do not migrate normally in an inherited hypogonadal (Kallmann) syndrome. *Molecular Brain Research,* 1989;6(4):311-26.

[14] Valdes-Socin H., Almanza M. R., Fernández-Ladreda M. T., Debray F. G., Bours V., Beckers A. Reproduction, smell, and neurodevelopmental disorders: genetic defects in different hypogonadotropic hypogonadal syndromes. Frontiers in endocrinology. 2014; 5.

[15] Greydanus D. E., Omar H., Pratt H. D. The adolescent female athlete: current concepts and conundrums. *Pediatric Clinics of North America,* 2010; 57(3):697-718.

[16] De Souza M., Toombs R. Amenorrhea Associated With the Female Athlete Triad: Etiology, Diagnosis, and Treatment. Amenorrhea: Springer; 2010. p. 101-25.

[17] Roberto C. A., Steinglass J., Mayer L. E., Attia E., Walsh B. T. The clinical significance of amenorrhea as a diagnostic criterion for anorexia nervosa. *International Journal of Eating Disorders*, 2008; 41(6):559-63.

[18] McGarry K. A., Tong I. L. The 5-minute Consult Clinical Companion to Women's Health: Lippincott Williams and Wilkins; 2012.

[19] Bachelot A., Binart N. Reproductive role of prolactin. *Reproduction,* 2007; 133(2):361-9.

[20] Arnaldi G., Angeli A., Atkinson A., Bertagna X., Cavagnini F., Chrousos G., et al. Diagnosis and complications of Cushing's syndrome: a consensus statement. *The Journal of Clinical Endocrinology and Metabolism,* 2003; 88(12):5593-602.

[21] Master-Hunter T., Heiman D. L. Amenorrhea: evaluation and treatment. *Women*, 2006; 100(1):18.

[22] Di Pasquale E., Beck-Peccoz P., Persani L. Hypergonadotropic ovarian failure associated with an inherited mutation of human bone morphogenetic protein-15 (BMP15) gene. *The American Journal of Human Genetics,* 2004; 75(1):106-11.

[23] Sherman S. L. Premature ovarian failure in the fragile X syndrome. *American journal of medical genetics*, 2000; 97(3):189-94.

[24] Behtash N., Karimi Zarchi M. Dysgerminoma in three patients with Swyer syndrome. *World J. Surg. Oncol.*, 2007; 5(7).

[25] Whitaker K. N. Polycystic Ovary Syndrome An Overview. *Journal of pharmacy practice,* 2011;24(1):94-101.

[26] Parikh R. M., Nakum K., Kadikar G., Gokhle A. Mullerian anomalies: A cause of primary amenorrhea. *International J. Reproduction Contraception Obstet. Gynaecol.*, 2013; 2(3):393.

[27] New M. I. An update of congenital adrenal hyperplasia. *Annals of the New York Academy of Sciences,* 2004;1038(1):14-43.

In: Amenorrhea
Editor: Oliver Chukwujekwu Ezechi
ISBN: 978-1-63484-778-0

Chapter 6

TESTICULAR FEMINIZATION SYNDROME

Christian Chigozie Makwe
Department of Obstetrics and Gynaecology, Faculty of Clinical Sciences, College of Medicine, University of Lagos, Lagos, Nigeria

ABSTRACT

Testicular feminization syndrome properly known as complete androgen insensitivity syndrome (CAIS) is an inherited X-linked recessive condition with a mutation in the androgen receptor gene. CAIS is the consequence of an end-organ resistance to androgens. In this condition, chromosomally male (46 XY) individuals develop female external genitalia with blindly ending vagina but lack uterus and fallopian tubes. The gonads are testes with normal production of androgens and anti-mullerian hormone (AMH). All mullerian-derived structures are absent because the AMH inhibits mullerian development. At puberty, the increasing levels of androgens are converted to estrogens with normal female breast development and distribution of body fat. Affected individuals usually present with primary amenorrhea in adolescence but sometimes an inguinal mass or hernia maybe discovered at an early age. The standard of care consists of both medical and surgical interventions. Treatment aims to minimize potential psychosocial issues, improve sexual health, prevent gonadal malignancy and reduce risk of osteoporosis.

Keywords: testicular feminization syndrome, amenorrhea, fetal development

INTRODUCTION

Amenorrhea is the absence or abnormal cessation of menses [1]. Amenorrhea is a normal physiologic occurrence in prepubertal females. During puberty, normal menstruation depends on an intact hypothalamic-pituitary system, a functional ovary secreting ovarian hormones, a responsive endometrium and a patent outflow tract. Primary amenorrhea refers to a failure of spontaneous menstruation by the age of 16 years in the presence of normal secondary sexual characteristics, or 14 years in the absence of secondary sexual characteristics. Ideally, the age limit for defining primary amenorrhea is two standard deviations above the population mean age at menarche [1]. Primary amenorrhea is often, but not exclusively, the result of disorders of sex development (DSDs) such as complete gonadal dysgenesis, Mullerian agenesis and complete androgen insensitivity syndrome (formerly known as testicular feminization syndrome). DSDs are congenital conditions in which anatomical, chromosomal or gonadal sex is atypical [2].

Testicular feminization syndrome was first fully described by Dr. John Morris, an American gynaecologist, in 1953 [3]. He described the entity in 82 cases collected from medical literature. All were phenotypic females with 46XY karyotype, presenting with primary amenorrhea, adequate breast development, and absent or scanty pubic and axillary hairs. Morris coined the term "testicular feminization syndrome" based on his observation that the testes in these individuals produced an estrogen-like hormone that caused feminization of the body. The syndrome has been called Morris syndrome in honour of Dr. John Morris [4].

Since 1953, scientists have carried out animal and human studies to elucidate the aetiopathogenesis of this condition. In 1970, researchers identified an X-linked gene for testicular feminization (Tfm) in mouse and established the X-chromosomal localization of the Tfm locus [5]. In 1981, Migeon et al. reported the localization of the androgen receptor locus on the human X chromosome and the evidence for homology with the Tfm locus in the mouse [6]. In 1989, the exact localization of the human Androgen Receptor (AR) gene on Xq11-12 was defined by Brown et al. [7]. Further genetic studies proved that mutations in the AR gene causes androgen insensitivity syndrome [8-10].

Androgen insensitivity syndrome (AIS) is an inherited X-linked recessive condition caused by mutations in the AR gene. AIS can be classified into three phenotypes: complete AIS (CAIS), partial AIS (PAIS) and mild AIS (MAIS). Theoretically, it is possible for AIS to occur in individuals with 46XX karyotype (homozygote) but the clinical manifestations only occur in individuals with 46XY karyotype (heterozygote).

PATHOGENESIS

Androgen Receptor Gene and the Androgen Receptor

The AR gene is a single copy gene that spans approximately 90kb of genomic DNA and the AR gene locus is on proximal long arm of X chromosome (Xq11-12). The protein coding region consists of 8 exons and separated by introns [11]. The exons code for a protein that has 3 main functional domains: N-terminal domain (NTD or transactivation domain); DNA binding domain (DBD); and the ligand-binding domain (LBD). Exon 1 encodes for the NTD. Within exon 1, the repetitions of the glutamine codon (CAG) and glycine codon (GGC) are highly polymorphic in length. Exons 2-3 encodes for the DBD. Exons 4 to 8 encode for LBD.

AR is a member of the nuclear receptor superfamily that functions as a ligand-activated transcription factor. The AR mediates the biological activity of androgens and it is expressed in fetal tissues as early as 8 weeks of gestation. AR protein consists of approximately 919 aminoacids. The AR is organized in 3 main functional domains. The NTD comprises of 557 aminoacids and regulates target gene transcription. The DBD consists of 70 aminoacids and is highly conserved with two zinc finger modules. DBD determines the specificity of AR interaction with DNA. When bound to DNA, the DBD shows two zinc finger modules whose structure is dependent on cysteine interaction with zinc ion [12]. One zinc finger module structure is involved in specific recognition of the androgen-response element and direct DNA-binding; while the other is implicated in protein-protein interactions and serves as a stabilization unit of the dimerization of the two molecules [13]. The LBD comprises of 12 α-helices and 4 short β-strands arranged in a typical α-helical sandwich. A ligand-binding pocket, formed from the α-helical structure, provides an interaction surface for proteins such as co-activators and co-repressors [13, 14]. The main function of LBD is specific high-affinity binding of androgens. The LBD is also involved in nuclear localization, receptor dimerization and interaction with other proteins [13].

Androgens and Mechanism of Action

Androgens are produced mainly from the adrenal glands, the gonads (testes and ovaries), and peripheral sites such as skin, fat, liver and genitourinary system. Testosterone and its biologically active metabolite dihydrotestosterone (DHT) are the only androgens with direct androgenic effect. DHT is a more potent androgen derived from testosterone by the action of 5-alpha reductase enzyme in target tissues such as external genitalia, hair follicle and sebaceous gland.

Androgen enters the cell by simple diffusion through the cell membrane. Testosterone or DHT binds and activates the AR in the cytoplasm to form a ligand-AR complex. The hormone-activated AR complex undergoes conformational change and translocates to the nucleus; where dimerization, DNA binding and recruitment of coactivator occurs. Target genes are transcribed (mRNA) and translated into proteins [15-18].

The biological action of androgen occurs in a variety of tissues with ARs such as genitourinary tract, skin, fat, gastrointestinal tract, skeletal muscles, bone and brain.

Fetal Sex Development

Normal fetal sex development involves sex determination and sex differentiation. At conception, chromosomal (genetic) sex is determined based on whether the ovum is fertilized by X-chromosome sperm or Y-chromosome sperm. Normally, genetic male embryos have 46 XY karyotype and genetic female embryos have 46XX karyotypes. In normal sex differentiation, genetic sex determines gonadal sex and gonadal sex determines phenotypic sex.

Sex differentiation involves gonadal differentiation (development of undifferentiated bipotential gonad into either a testis or an ovary), differentiation of the internal ducts and differentiation of the external genitalia. The entire process of sex differentiation extends from fetal life to adulthood, and depends on the appropriate and timely interaction of several factors such as genes, proteins, hormones and paracrine factors. The accurate timing of normal testosterone synthesis or normal androgen responsiveness is essential for normal internal and/or external genital differentiation.

At about 4 to 5 weeks of gestation, the bipotential primitive gonad arises from a condensation of the mesoderm at the medioventral region of the urogenital ridge. Before 8 weeks of gestation, genetic male and female fetuses are "anatomically indistinguishable." The embryo has a pair undifferentiated bipotential gonad and two pairs of accessory sex ducts: the Wolffian ducts and the Mullerian ducts. At about 8 weeks of gestation, the bipotential gonad progresses toward testis organogenesis in the presence of testis-determining factor (TDF) gene. The TDF gene is located on the sex-determining region of Y chromosome (SRY). In the absence of TDF genes or SRY, the bipotential gonad develops into an ovary.

The testis is the primary source of androgen during fetal life. In the presence of functioning testis, testosterone and anti-mullerian hormone (AMH) are produced by Leydig cells and Sertoli cells respectively. The development of the internal ducts results from the paracrine effect of the ipsilateral gonad. Testosterone induces the Wolffian duct to develop into epididymis, vas deferens, and seminal vesicles. AMH induces regression of the Mullerian duct. The external genitalia differentiate towards the male phenotype under the influence of DHT. The genital tubercle, genital folds and genital swelling differentiate into the glans penis, penile shaft and scrotum, respectively. The prostate gland develops from the urogenital sinus under the androgenic effect of DHT.

In the absence of testicular tissue, the internal ducts and the external genitalia develop towards the female phenotype. The absence of AMH results in the development of Mullerian-derived structures: fallopian tubes, uterus, cervix and upper part of the vaginal. The Wolffian duct degenerates in the absence of testicular androgen. In the absence of androgen, the genital tubercle, genital folds and genital swelling differentiate into the clitoris, labia minor and labia major respectively.

Molecular Pathogenesis of CAIS

Mutation of AR gene causes CAIS and more than 95% of affected individuals have mutation of the AR [12]. Over 800 mutations have been described, including complete or partial gene deletions, nucleotide insertions or deletions, duplications, and single point mutations. AR mutations (pathogenic variants) may result in severe or significant functional defects due to the following: complete absence of AR; incomplete protein synthesis; altered androgen-receptor binding affinity or post-receptor signal abnormalities. Pathogenic variants of the AR mutation are distributed throughout the eight exons of the AR gene, but localized mainly in the LBD and the DBD [12].

In CAIS, the basic pathophysiology is a complete loss-of-function of AR. During fetal life, genetically male individuals with normal testis determination and androgen production fail to develop male internal duct and external genitalia because of end-organs resistant to androgens. The AMH produced by the Sertoli cells of testes inhibit the development of all Mullerian-derived structures. At birth, affected individuals have normal female external genitalia with a short vagina that ends blindly. The fallopian tubes, uterus and cervix are absent. During puberty, the testes under the influence of pituitary gonadotropins produce increasing levels of androgens which are converted to estrogens by aromatization. The estrogen leads to normal female breast development and distribution of body fat. The individual resembles a normal adult female, except for the almost complete absence of pubic and axillary hair.

EPIDEMIOLOGY

CAIS is a rare condition. The incidence has been estimated to be between 1 in 20,400 and 1 in 99,100 male births [19]. About two-thirds of all cases are inherited from the mothers who carry a pathogenic AR gene (heterozygote); while the remaining cases result from de novo mutation in the ovum before conception or in early embryonic life. In females who are carriers, their male children have a 50% chance of being affected while their female children have a 50% chance of being a carrier. A woman with an affect child has a 25% risk of recurrence in subsequent pregnancy. No racial or ethnic difference has been described for CAIS.

CLINICAL PRESENTATION

Patient with Testicular feminization syndrome present typically with primary amenorrhea in apparently normal female with good breast development. Other clinical features include inguinal or labial swelling, Lack of pubic and axillary hair, painful intercourse as a result of short vagina and infertility.

The patient may also presents with complication of the condition which include psychological and social issues, testicular malignancy, osteoporosis and complication of hormone replacement therapy.

DIAGNOSIS

Diagnosis of this condition is usually through clinical findings, hormonal assay, genetic analysis, and radiological imaging.

History and Physical Examination

In newborn, the external genitalia have the appearance of normal female and most frequently the presence of unilateral or bilateral inguinal mass (testis). The testes may be located in the labia or abdomen or within a hernia sac. The undescended testis may or may not be associated with hernias. There may be a history of an older sibling with inguinal mass or surgery.

Adolescent patients usually present with primary amenorrhea. There may be a history of prior surgery for hernia or inguinal mass at an early age. A positive family history of primary amenorrhea may be obtained from an older sibling. Physical examination reveals normal breast development, absent or scanty pubic and axillary hairs. Genital examination reveals a normal external female genitalia and a short vagina that ends blindly. The uterus and fallopian tube are absent. The testes may be present in the labia or inguinal canal. Later in life, affected individuals may present with coital difficulties and/or primary infertility.

Hormonal Assay

In Infants, a marked elevation of serum testosterone induced by luteinizing hormone (LH) surge occurs in males compared to females during the first few months of life (0-3 months). Following this LH-induced testosterone elevation, serum gonadotropins and testosterone remains low until puberty.

In women with CAIS, serum testosterone and LH estimations are within or above the normal range for males. Serum estradiol concentrations are higher than the values in males but lower than the estimate in normal (46XX) females. Follicular stimulating hormone and inhibin concentrations are generally normal.

Genetic Analysis

Chromatin analysis shows that individuals with male (XY) karyotype have negative sex chromatin on buccal mucosa smear. Chromosomal analysis will confirm the individual's karyotype as 46 XY. The presence of Y chromosome can also be confirmed by fluorescence in situ hybridization (FISH). The turnaround time for FISH is shorter compared to conventional karyotype. Molecular genetic testing can detect various types (pathogenic variants) of AR gene mutation. The methods available for genetic testing include sequence analysis, linkage analysis, deletion analysis and duplication analysis.

Androgen Binding Assay

This in-vitro assay measures AR binding in fibroblast obtained from genital skin (scrotal, foreskin or labial tissues). Genital skin fibroblast has a high concentration of ARs. In CAIS, androgen binding is typically absent.

Radiological Imaging

Pelvic ultrasonography reveals the absence of uterus and may be helpful in the localization of the gonads (testes). Magnetic resonance imaging and computerized tomography are alternative imaging techniques. Magnetic resonance imaging appears to be most useful in localizing the gonads and planning for surgery.

Testicular Biopsy

In infants or prepubertal girls, biopsy of the gonads may be performed to confirm the presence of testicular tissue on histopathology. Testicular biopsy shows immature germ cells with atrophic seminiferous tubules and hyperplastic Leydig cells.

Laparoscopy or Laparotomy

Diagnostic laparoscopy or exploratory laparotomy with biopsy of the intra-abdominal gonads may be indicated in certain clinical settings, where it is difficult to establish a diagnosis. The absence of uterus and fallopian tubes will be confirmed at surgery.

Management

The management of CAIS is currently limited to symptomatic management as no management strategy is currently available to correct the malfunctioning androgen receptor proteins produced by the AR gene mutations. The options of management include genetic counselling, psychological counselling, hormone replacement therapy, vaginoplasty and gonadectomy.

A multidisciplinary team is required to provide effective diagnosis, treatment and support care. The team usually consists of geneticist, genetic counselor, paediatric endocrinologist, clinical psychologist, psychiatrist, gynaecologist and surgeon.

At birth, individuals with CAIS are unequivocally assigned female gender identity and sex of rearing. There has not been any reported female to male gender conversion at puberty.

Genetic Counselling

Genetic counselling and psychological support are essential components of medical care. The parents of an affected child and an affected older individual should be adequately counselled on the nature of the condition, the mode of inheritance and the need to identify other potential carriers in the family.

Psychological Counselling and Support

The parents of an affected child and affected older individuals should be counselled on the treatment modalities including all personal, cultural and ethical issues they may encounter. Parents should have the knowledge and skills required to educate the child about the condition in an age-appropriate manner. An affected older individual should also have gender and sexual counselling.

Medical experts should also provide psychological support services including linkage to support groups. An affected older individual may develop significant psychosocial issues such gender identity issues, self-doubts, social isolation, anger, and depression. Adequate psychological counselling and support services may help ameliorate these potential problems.

Following genetic screening, any other affected family member or carrier should be counselled appropriately and given the necessary psychological support.

Hormone Replacement Therapy

Hormone replacement therapy (HRT) is advised following surgical removal of the testes (orchidectomy) in adolescent or young adult patients. Individuals with CAIS have reduced mineral bone density and increased risk of fractures [20]. In CAIS, HRT invariably means estrogen replacement. Estrogen therapy induces and maintains feminization of the affected individual, and prevents the long-term risk of osteoporosis. Evidence suggests that progestogen administration may have little or no advantage in individuals without uterus. However, long-term estrogen therapy may be associated with an increases risk of breast cancer.

Gonadectomy

Orchidectomy is performed to prevent possible malignant transformation and development of gonadoblastoma of the testes. Most recently, postpubertal orchidectomy is preferred to prepubertal orchidectomy. The rationale for postpubertal orchidectomy is the fact that testicular malignancy rarely occur before puberty, and testicular steroids are necessary for complete feminization of the affected individual. In the past, prepubertal orchidectomy was performed to avoid psychosexual issues that may develop during adolescence and young adulthood. At present, prepubertal orchidectomy may only be justified when the inguinal testis causes significant discomfort or as a concurrent procedure during inguinal herniorrhaphy.

Vaginoplasty

Vaginal dilatation to augment vaginal length is recommended for those with short vaginal length. This aims to avoid dyspareunia and ensure satisfactory penetrative vaginal intercourse with partner. Alternatively, a neovagina may be created through autologous graft such as buccal mucosa graft vaginoplasty and peritoneum vaginoplasty or enhance balloon vaginoplasty. The use of vaginal dilators is encouraged to prevent vaginal stenosis following vaginoplasty. Vaginal lengthening procedures are best performed when sexual debut is imminent.

Delaying surgery until the affected individual is sufficiently mature to participate actively in the decision-making process is advocated by many support groups. At an appropriate age with a fully informed consent, the affected individual can have the surgical procedures (orchidectomy, inguinal herniorrhaphy, and vaginoplasty) performed at the same time.

Management of Infertility

Occasionally, the diagnosis of CAIS is first established during evaluation for primary infertility. Individuals with CAIS lack both uterus and ovaries. Affected individuals should be adequately counselled on the available treatment options such as adoption, assisted conception with gestational surrogate and oocyte donation or following uterine transplantation.

Following in-vitro fertilization, embryo formed using male partner's sperm and donor oocyte is transferred to a gestational surrogate. A recent report of livebirth following uterine transplantation and in-vitro fertilization has expanded the reproductive options available to women with congenital absence of the uterus [21].

Prevention

Prevention of AIS revolves around the identification of women who may carry the gene and the provision of appropriate nondirective counselling and genetic testing. Genetic counselling and testing should be offered to at-risk relatives of an affected individual to identify women who are carriers.

Preconception care provides opportunity for clarification of carrier status of the woman and determination of genetic risk before pregnancy. Women who carry pathogenic AR mutations should be offered preconception counselling including genetic counselling. This allows them to make an informed decision about whether to have children or not.

Pregnant women who carry pathogenic variants of the AR mutation may be offered prenatal diagnosis. Chorionic villous sampling and amniocentesis can be performed to obtain sample for karyotyping. The diagnosis of CAIS may be suspected when discordance exists in sex identified by karyotype (XY) and ultrasonography (female).

Pre-implantation genetic diagnosis may be offered to couples undergoing in-vitro fertilization and embryo transfer, where the female partner has been identified as a carrier of pathogenic AR mutation.

Prognosis

The prognosis is excellent in women with CAIS, if gonadectomy is performed at the right time with appropriate support and counselling. Optimal management of affected older individual has led to satisfactory sexual life and the possibility now exists for uterine-transplant births.

Conclusion

Individuals with CAIS should receive long-term, multidisplinary, client-centered care. The clinical considerations of therapy should be to minimize potential psychosocial issues, maximize client's decision-making, improve sexual health and prevent gonadal malignancy.

References

[1] Current evaluation of amenorrhea. *Fertility and sterility* 2008;90:S219-25.

[2] Barno A. Testicular feminization syndrome in male pseudohermaphrodites. *American journal of obstetrics and gynecology* 1962;84:710-8.

[3] Morris JM. The syndrome of testicular feminization in male pseudohermaphrodites. *American journal of obstetrics and gynecology* 1953;65:1192-211.

[4] Brinkmann OA, Griehl A, Kuwertz-Broking E, Bulla M, Hertle L. Extracorporeal shock wave lithotripsy in children. Efficacy, complications and long-term follow-up. *European urology* 2001;39:591-7.

[5] Lyon MF, Hawkes SG. X-linked gene for testicular feminization in the mouse. *Nature* 1970;227:1217-9.

[6] Hughes IA, Werner R, Bunch T, Hiort O. Androgen insensitivity syndrome. *Seminars in reproductive medicine* 2012;30:432-42.

[7] Das Gupta TK. Testicular feminisation. *Journal of the Indian Medical Association* 1966;47:333-5.

[8] Piver MS, Goldfarb AF, Rakoff AE, Traum R. Testicular feminization. A study of two families. *Obstetrics and gynecology* 1966;28:397-400.

[9] Philip J, Sele V. Testicular Feminization. (Karyotypic-Linkage and Endocrine Studies in Three Sibs with the Complete Syndrome). A*cta endocrinologica* 1965;48:297-312.

[10] Ijzerman A, Gerards JJ. [a Case of Testicular Feminization]. *Nederlandsch tijdschrift voor verloskunde en gynaecologie* 1963;63:261-8.

[11] Marcelli M, Tilley WD, Wilson CM, Griffin JE, Wilson JD, McPhaul MJ. Definition of the human androgen receptor gene structure permits the identification of mutations that cause androgen resistance: premature termination of the receptor protein at amino acid residue 588 causes complete androgen resistance. *Mol Endocrinol* 1990;4:1105-16.

[12] Hughes IA, Davies JD, Bunch TI, Pasterski V, Mastroyannopoulou K, MacDougall J. Androgen insensitivity syndrome. *Lancet* 2012;380: 1419-28.

[13] Galani A, Kitsiou-Tzeli S, Sofokleous C, Kanavakis E, Kalpini-Mavrou A. Androgen insensitivity syndrome: clinical features and molecular defects. *Hormones* (Athens) 2008;7:217-29.

[14] Matias PM, Donner P, Coelho R, et al. Structural evidence for ligand specificity in the binding domain of the human androgen receptor. Implications for pathogenic gene mutations. *The Journal of biological chemistry* 2000;275:26164-71.

[15] Quigley CA, De Bellis A, Marschke KB, el-Awady MK, Wilson EM, French FS. Androgen receptor defects: historical, clinical, and molecular perspectives. *Endocrine reviews* 1995;16:271-321.

[16] Gottlieb B, Lombroso R, Beitel LK, Trifiro MA. Molecular pathology of the androgen receptor in male (in)fertility. *Reproductive biomedicine online* 2005;10:42-8.

[17] Choong CS, Wilson EM. Trinucleotide repeats in the human androgen receptor: a molecular basis for disease. *Journal of molecular endocrinology* 1998;21:235-57.

[18] Meehan KL, Sadar MD. Androgens and androgen receptor in prostate and ovarian malignancies. Frontiers in bioscience: *A journal and virtual library* 2003;8:d780-800.

[19] Boehmer AL, Brinkmann O, Bruggenwirth H, et al. Genotype versus phenotype in families with androgen insensitivity syndrome. *The Journal of clinical endocrinology and metabolism* 2001;86:4151-60.

[20] Oakes MB, Eyvazzadeh AD, Quint E, Smith YR. Complete androgen insensitivity syndrome--a review. *Journal of pediatric and adolescent gynecology* 2008;21:305-10.

[21] Brannstrom M, Diaz-Garcia C, Johannesson L, Dahm-Kahler P, Bokstrom H. Livebirth after uterus transplantation - Authors' reply. *Lancet* 2015;385:2352-3.

In: Amenorrhea
Editor: Oliver Chukwujekwu Ezechi
ISBN: 978-1-63484-778-0

Chapter 7

ANDROGEN INSENSITIVITY SYNDROME

Odidika Ugochukwu Joannes Umeora[1] and Maryjoanne Chinyem Umeora[2]
[1]Department of Obstetrics and Gynaecology, Ebonyi State University Abakaliki, Nigeria
[2]Department of Pediatrics, Newark-Beth Israel Children's hospital, New Jersey, US

ABSTRACT

Androgen Insensitivity Syndrome is a rare but exciting spectrum of pathology involving some form of a disconnect between the genetic makeup of an individual and his phenotypic appearance. Complete understanding of the aetiology of this syndrome may be lacking but AR gene located on the long arm of the X chromosome has been implicated and is transmitted in an x-linked fashion with variable penetrance. The individuals have a 46XY genetic makeup but demonstrate various forms of end organ resistance to the male hormone. Three variants of complete Androgen Insensitivity Syndrome, Partial Androgen Insensitivity Syndrome and Mild Androgen Insensitivity Syndrome are recognised. Diagnosis is based on history, physical examination and investigations. Management requires multidisciplinary approach involving the endocrinologist, paediatrician, gynaecologist urologist and clinical psychologist. This condition runs in families and relatives can be put under surveillance especially in families where the pathogenic AR gene has been documented.

Keywords: Androgen Insenstivity Syndrome, amenorrhea, fertilization

INTRODUCTION

Primary amenorrhea constitutes a source of anxiety and worry to not just the individual but also her parents and care givers. Critical evaluation comprising history, physical examination and investigations becomes necessary for optimal management. An important aetiological factor is Androgen Insensitivity Syndrome (AIS) which is a 46XY disorder of sex development (DSD).

After fertilization the human zygote possesses a bipotential gonad. Definitive differentiation of the gonad depends entirely on the presence or absence of the testicular differentiating factor (TDF). The Y sex chromosome only, bears the TDF which controls development of the Wolffian structures and male internal and external sex structures, via elaboration of age appropriate amounts of androgens. In the absence of TDF, the default sex, female persists. The final development of the male phenotype not only depends on adequate amount of androgens but also on adequate response to it by the end organs. Resistance to the androgens may result in abnormalities in the reproductive tract [1]. In Androgen insensitivity syndrome (AIS), there is a varying degree of resistance of the end organs resulting in a spectrum of external sex abnormalities. In complete AIS (CAIS) the XY individual with testes and no Müllerian structures like the uterus and Fallopian tubes presents phenotypically as a female. In some (about 30%), however, the Müllerian structures do not regress completely leaving some Müllerian remnants [2]. Some Wolffian structures like epididymides, vasa deferentia and seminal vesicles are typically absent or partially developed in a third of cases [3]. For this it was erroneously referred to as testicular feminization syndrome but recently complete Androgen insensitivity syndrome (CAIS) which is more appropriate [4].

In other manifestations due to partial resistance (PAIS) the XY individual presents with different degrees of abnormalities which may be mostly male or mostly female. The mild form (MAIS) may proceed unnoticed till puberty when the individual develops undue gynaecomastia or presents with infertility. It is this apparent varying presentation stretching from infancy to adulthood that makes this syndrome unique and requires a clear understanding by physicians, parents and patients alike.

Complete Androgen Insensitivity Syndrome (CAIS)

As the name implies, there is total resistance to the hormone at the end organ targets, this unresponsiveness to circulating androgens prevents masculinization of the fetal genitalia in utero and development of male secondary sexual characteristics at puberty. But this resistance in no way alters the genetic makeup. The gonads are testes since these develop from an androgen-independent process owing to the presence of SRY gene on the Y chromosome [5, 6]. These may be found intra-abdominally, at the inguinal region or labia majora. As such, ultrasonographic findings or other prenatal investigations including karyotyping, chorionic villus sampling, amniotic fluid analysis and maternal free fetal DNA analysis may conflict with apparent sex at birth [7]. Furthermore, there may be a family history of same (X-linked). These individuals at birth are almost of same size as normal males showing that the control may be located on the Y chromosome [8]. They subsequently grow taller than females without the syndrome but on the average shorter than their male counterparts. A red herring that appears is the presence of bilateral inguinal hernia or labial swelling in such females. Bilateral inguinal hernias are ordinarily rare in females. A biopsy of gonads found in the swelling for karyotyping should be undertaken following parental permission [9]. Physical examination will reveal a short vagina following absence of the upper vagina, cervix and uterus, all derivable from the Müllerian duct which regresses in the presence of Müllerian Inhibitory Factor (MIF) occasioned by the Y sex chromosome [10]. These individuals commence pubertal changes at the appropriate age or a bit delayed often with breast buds and growth spurts, however, axillary and pubic hair are scanty or may be absent, menarche is never achieved. Primary amenorrhea may be the first presentation in many. Hormonal assay will yield normal or high levels of testosterone for men or boys and a much higher levels of luteinizing hormone. Estrogens derived from peripheral aromatization of androgens and from the gonads are higher than in males but lower than in females without the syndrome [11]. In infancy, the serum testosterone level is low in affected infants but the anti Müllerian hormone is higher than in normal males [12].

Because of the primary amenorrhea, differential diagnoses would include complete gonadal dysgenesis (but these patients would not have high AMH), Mayer-Rokitansky-Kuster-Hauser syndrome and Transverse vaginal septum amongst other causes of primary amenorrhea.

Partial Androgen Insensitivity Syndrome (PAIS)

Partial Androgen Insensitivity Syndrome (PAIS) presents with different degrees of undermasculinization as well as near female phenotype depending on the degree of the end organs' response to circulating androgens. In PAIS, the degree of androgen insensitivity leads to partial masculinization of the genitalia but not enough to completely prevent it [13, 14]. In the severe form (almost resembling CAIS) the individual is almost female but for the degree of clitoromegaly. In the almost male form, there is micropenis with severe hypospadias and occasional bifid scrotum which may contain the testes. Quigley et al. [4] proposed seven grades of PAIS as follows - grades 1 through 6 distinguished by the extent of genital masculinization; grade 1 indicates fully masculinized external genitalia and grade 6 when the external genitalia is almost fully feminized, and grades 2 through 5 refer to four degrees of increasingly feminized genitalia that lie within the spectrum. Grade 7 is indistinguishable from grade 6 until puberty, and is thereafter differentiated by the presence of secondary terminal hair (grade 6) or its absence (grade 7). Unlike in CAIS, Wolffian structures like the epididymides, seminal vesicles and vasa differentia are either partially or fully developed [13], the prostate is present too but rudimentary [15, 16]. Mullerian remnants are rare [17, 18]. Risk of germ cell tumour is more than that obtains in cases of CAIS with reported rate of about 15% especially when the testes are found anywhere but intrascrotally [19]. In another report, the risk was documented as up to 50% in undescended testes [20]. The AR gene mutation associated with PAIS has also been linked to cancer of the breast and prostate [21-24].

Diagnosis of PAIS requires extensive investigation to exclude differentials like pure gonadal dysgenesis, enzyme deficiencies (5 alpha reductase 2, 17,20-lyase, P450 oxidoreductase and 17β-hydroxysteroid dehydrogenase type 3) as well as genetic malformations as Klinefelter's syndrome, Denys-Drash syndrome and Frasier's syndrome [11]. It is postulated that in PAIS the Androgen receptor (AR) gene may be defective or normal with fetal growth restriction [11].

Mild Androgen Insensitivity Syndrome (MAIS)

Defect in the AR gene has been implicated also in Mild Androgen insensitivity Syndrome (MAIS). The individuals are male without abnormalities in their genitalia [25] but presents with infertility. Some also present with spinal and bulbar muscular atrophy linked with expansion CAG repeats in the AR gene [26]. The latter present with muscle wasting and weakness as well as gynaecomastia, infertility and high androgen levels consistent with PAIS.

PATHOGENESIS

The key to understanding AIS lies in understanding the AR gene which has been implicated in its aetiology. The AR gene is located on chromosome X at the Xq [11-12] loci [27, 28]. They are nuclear receptors and are activated by either testosterone or dihydrotestosterone (DHT) [29] and act via gene transcription. Androgen-regulated genes are vital for the development and preservation of male phenotypic structures and appearance. Therefore adequate response to androgens is needed for the development of the phallus as well as the scrotum in the male. This is lacking in CAIS and suboptimal in PAIS and MAIS. However, there is normal conversion of testosterone to dihydrotestosterone in AIS and this differentiates it from 5 alpha reductase deficiency. The AR gene also referred to as NR3C4 (Nuclear receptor, subfamily 3, group C member 4) is modulated by acetylation. In AIS there are defects in this gene via point mutation or trinucleotide repeats polymorphism amongst others [30]. The point mutations are mainly mis-sense distributed throughout the eight axons on the AR gene [31]. Over 1,000 such mutations have been documented, including complete and partial gene deletions, small insertion/deletions and point mutations. These mutations lead to a variety of functional defects, ranging from a total loss of receptors on the cell surface because of incomplete protein synthesis to alterations in substrate binding affinity. Altered substrate binding affinity causes a signal transmission loss, despite normal cell surface receptor numbers [32]. Transmission is in X-linked recessive fashion [13, 33]. Mutations are found in about 95% of CAIS while the rate of spontaneous mutation is about 30% which approximates that in other X-linked disorders like haemophilia [11]. The mutation occurs mainly at the ligand-binding domain. The androgen receptors are prevalent in genital skin fibroblasts and biopsy of these can give a clue to the pathology encountered in AIS. In CAIS, androgen binding is noticeably absent and attenuated in PAIS and MAIS [34].

In a few percentage, no mutation is observed in the AR gene. In such individuals, mutant steroidogenic factor 1 (SF-1) [35] and a transactivating signalling defect involving the N-terminal region of the normal AR receptors [36] have been implicated.

MANAGEMENT

AIS presents with complex management challenge whenever and in whatever forms it manifests. At varying stages, it poses gynaecological, neonatological, urological, surgical and endocrinological challenge, implying that a multidisciplinary approach to management involving these specialists is apt. In addition, needed would be clinical psychologists, social workers, ethicists, and sexual therapists/genetic counsellors amongst others to manage the attendant psychosocial, ethical and sexual concerns. Because of the varying presentation also and individualised needs, management needs to be tailored and holistic and involving the family in most cases. No rigid regimen or protocol need be upheld as flexible schedule may provide better management outcome. In-depth knowledge of other disorders of sex developments is also necessary for appropriate management which depends on the severity and individual manifestation of the AIS.

At birth, CAIS hardly poses any problems as the individual is often assigned a female sex of rearing except when earlier prenatal sex suggestion contrasts the phenotype at birth. This should prompt rigorous evaluations along the line of DSDs to make a diagnosis. More commonly a female presenting with bilateral inguinal hernia is assessed by gonadal biopsy following parental consent. And where biopsy is positive for CAIS, it raises the issue of necessity and timing for gonadectomy. It is believed that the gonads may develop malignant germ cell tumour and hence the need for gonadectomy. The Australian Paediatric Endocrine group believes that this risk is minimal and hence did not recommend routine gonadectomy, rather patients should be monitored for this regularly [37]. The risk is generally put at approximately 2% [20]. The risk is however known to increase with age getting to 3.6% by 25 years and 32% at 50 years [38]. It is rare before puberty [3], a rate of 0.8% was reported [13]. Gonadectomy may be performed before puberty which would now be induced using Estrogen replacement therapy [13]. In most cases gonadectomy is performed post puberty. Whenever this is done, ERT remains essential to prevent osteoporosis in later life [39-40]. In the absence of an uterus, there is no fear for development of endometrial cancer on ERT, progestin replacement is not necessary, however, androgen replacement has been shown to increase the feeling well-being in individuals with gonadectomy (Hughes 2006) [13]. Further surgical intervention may be needed to create a neovagina or improve upon the capacity of an existing one, especially when this is short to allow for satisfactory sexual function. These are however better undertaken when non surgical methods like vaginal dilators have failed [41].

From the time of diagnosis through to management, psychological support for the parents and family and the individual is vital. Affected adolescents or young adults may lose self-esteem, feel anger, pain and rejection, may reject their status and react angrily to life and the world. The mothers on the other hand, may feel as sense of guilt and worthlessness having passed on the condition to their off springs. The need for professional counselling can therefore not be over emphasized. Clinical psychologists as well as child psychologists should be at hand to help the family go through disclosure to the minor or the affected adult depending on the age at diagnosis [13, 42]. They need to be supported throughout the acute management schedules and thereafter especially as they remain under health watch/monitoring for life. Prominent issues to be considered include pubertal changes, the presence of XY genotype and testes, potential for malignancy, surgery (gonadectomy/ vaginoplasty), sexual functions and infertility. Infertility amongst those already in union should be promptly addressed. They cannot conceive and therefore adoption or surrogacy using partner's semen in climes where this is legal may be an alternative [11].

Since it presents with genital sex ambiguities at birth, PAIS presents an earlier management challenge than does CAIS. Unfortunately, differentials for PAIS are myriad (Hughes 2006) [13]. A quick diagnosis is essential in a child with genital ambiguity, as some causes are associated with potentially life-threatening adrenal crises [5] testosterone, and dihydrotestosterone (DHT) assay at baseline and/or after human chorionic gonadotropin (hCG) stimulation can be used to exclude such defects in androgen biosynthesis [14]. Highlight of definitive management includes sex assignment, corrective surgery, gonadectomy and counselling. Grades 1 and 6 may be obviously male and female respectively but such certainty may not apply to the other grades especially 3 and 4. Indicated laboratory investigations and a multidisciplinary involvement at birth is encouraged for an expeditious sex assignment considering appearance of the genitalia [20] potential to virilize at puberty [14], surgical choices and the postoperative sexual function of the genitalia [43], potential for fertility [20] and the anticipated gender identity of the child [44]. The majority of individuals with PAIS are raised male [13]. Potential for virilisation can be assessed following response to exogenous androgens, genital skin fibroblasts and response to human chorionic gonadotropins [4]. All tests need be interpreted with caution.

The type, extent and timing of genitoplasty need to be individualized depending on the structures and/or malformation(s) involved as well as the assigned gender. Multiple surgical interventions may be required. Common recommendations in the males include repair of hypospadias and undescended testes at 2 to 3 years, reduction mammoplasty at puberty. Androgen supplementation may also be required at puberty. In the female, genitoplasty is encouraged before puberty.

Potential for malignancy is higher with PAIS so the need for gonadectomy. It is recommended that this operation be performed at the time of diagnosis if there is cryptochidism [20]. Prepubertal gonadectomy in the female will imply estrogen replacement therapy to induce female puberty. Induced puberty in this way also results in development of secondary sexual characteristics, growth spurt and bone mineral accumulation [20]. Women with PAIS may have a tendency towards osteoporosis but at a degree less than that in CAIS, and is similarly managed [45].

The psychological morbidity attending PAIS appears more profound than that in CAIS. Some patients may be dysphoric concerning their genitalia and have concerns about sexual functions, intimate relationships, fertility and acceptance by the society. Psychological support from infancy, through adolescence to adulthood is necessary. It means once again that child psychologists as well as clinical psychologists and genetic counsellors form part of the multidisciplinary management team.

Individuals with MAIS are males with male phenotype. In this condition response to androgens is mildly impaired to affect spermatogenesis and/or pubertal secondary sexual changes but not enough to impair differentiation and development of the genitals [4, 13, 14]. It is the least known and mildest form of AIS [25] It is estimated that 2-3% of infertile men have AR gene mutations [46]. MAIS may present with oligospermia or azoospermia [25, 47] mild gynaecomastia in young adulthood, decreased secondary terminal hair, high pitched voice, or minor hypospadias [11, 48]. The Wolffian structures (the epididymides, vasa deferentia, and seminal vesicles) and the prostate, are also normal. They have no Müllerian remnants. Suspicions of MAIS occur during evaluations for male infertility [42]. It is not easy distinguishing between men with and without MAIS, and thus a diagnosis of MAIS is usually made only with confirmation of an AR gene mutation [25]. A high Androgen sensitivity index (ASI) which is a product of Luteinizing hormone and Testosterone in a normal phenotypic male [49] especially with azoospermia or oligospermia [25, 47] decreased secondary terminal hair [50], can be indicative of MAIS. However in some cases of MAIS, ASI may be normal. Management of MAIS is mainly symptomatic. Some surgical procedures like mammoplasty for gynaecomastia and repair of hypospadias might be indicated. High levels of Testosterone may reverse oligospermia and help in treatment of infertility and correct impaired secondary sexual characteristics [20, 51]. For the associated link with breast and prostate cancers, regular monitoring for these is recommended [52, 53]. Psychological morbidity may arise from realisation of a diagnosis of AIS in however mild. Clinical psychologists have a vital role to play.

Conclusion

AIS in whatever degree presents an exciting spectrum of pathology to the clinician but to the affected and the family, it is a veritable source of anxiety, anxiety relating to phenotypic sex assignment, sex of rearing, sexual function, corrective surgeries, hormone replacement, fertility and fear of potential malignancy. The psychological and mental strain on the affected is enormous. While considering management options, a multidisciplinary approach is adopted and must include clinical psychologists and genetic counsellors. Long term follow up for potential germ cell malignancy, breast cancer and prostate cancer is advisable.

References

[1] Huhtaniemi I., Alevizaki M., Mutations along the hypothalamic-pituitary-gonadal axis affecting male reproduction. *Reprod Biomed Online* 2007; 15: 622–32.

[2] Nichols J. L., Bieber E. J., Gell J. S., Case of sisters with complete androgen insensitivity syndrome and discordant Müllerian remnants. *Fertil Steril.* 2009;91:932e15-e18.

[3] Hannema S. E., Scott I. S., Hodapp J., Martin H., Coleman N., Schwabe J. W., et al. "Residual activity of mutant androgen receptors explains wolffian duct development in the complete androgen insensitivity syndrome." *J. Clin. Endocrinol. Metab.* 2004; 89 (11): 5815–22.

[4] Quigley C. A., De Bellis A., Marschke K. B., el-Awady M. K., Wilson E. M., French F. S., Androgen receptor defects: historical, clinical, and molecular perspectives. *Endocr Rev* 1995; 16: 271–321.

[5] Achermann J. C., Jameson J. L., "Disorders of sexual differentiation." In Hauser S. L., Kasper D. L., Fauci A. S., Braunwald E., Longo D. L., Harrison's endocrinology. New York: *McGraw-Hill Medical Pub. Division* 2006. pp. 161–172.

[6] Simpson J. L., Rebar R. W., Hung, Wellington; Becker, Kenneth L.; Bilezikian, John P.; William J. Bremner, ed. Principles and Practice of Endocrinology and Metabolism. Hagerstwon, MD: *Lippincott Williams and Wilkins.* 2002; pp. 852–885.

[7] Yalinkaya A., Yayla M., Erdemoglu M., Prenatal diagnosis of a fetus with androgen insensitivity syndrome (AIS). *Prenat Diagn* 2007;27: 856–57.

[8] Miles H. L., Gidlof S., Nordenstrom A., Ong K. K., Hughes I. A., The role of androgens in fetal growth: observational study in two genetic models of disordered androgen signalling. *Arch Dis Child Fetal Neonatal E*d 2010; 95: F435–38.

[9] Winterborn M. H., France N. E., Raiti S., Incomplete testicular feminization. *Arch Dis Child.* 1970 Dec. 45(244):811-2.

[10] Hurme T., Lahdes-Vasama T., Makela E., Iber T., Toppari J., Clinical findings in prepubertal girls with inguinal hernia with special reference to the diagnosis of androgen insensitivity syndrome. *Scand J Urol Nephrol* 2009; 43: 42–46.

[11] Hughes I. A., Davies J. D., Bunch T. I., Pasterski, V., Mastroyannopoulou K., MacDougall J., Androgen Insensitivity. *Lancet* 2012 380: 1419–28.

[12] Rey R., Mebarki F., Forest M. G., et al. Anti-mullerian hormone in children with androgen insensitivity. *J Clin Endocrinol Metab* 1994; 79: 960–64.

[13] Hughes I. A., Deeb A., Androgen resistance. *Best Pract Res Clin Endocrinol Metab* 2006; 20: 577–98.

[14] Galani A., Kitsiou-Tzeli S., Sofokleous C., Kanavakis E., Kalpini-Mavrou. "Androgen insensitivity syndrome: clinical features and molecular defects." *Hormones* (Athens) 2008; 7 (3): 217–29.

[15] Boehmer A. L., Brinkmann O., Brüggenwirth H., van Assendelft C., Otten B. J., Verleun-Mooijman M. C., et al. Genotype versus phenotype in families with androgen insensitivity syndrome. *J Clin Endocrinol Metab* 2001; 86: 4151–60.

[16] Migeon C. J., Wisniewski A. B., Gearhart J. P., Meyer-Bahlburg H. F., Rock J. A., Brown T. R., et al. "Ambiguous genitalia with perineoscrotal hypospadias in 46,XY individuals: long-term medical, surgical, and psychosexual outcome." *Pediatrics* 2002; 110 (3): e31.

[17] Menakaya U. A., Aligbe J., Iribhogbe P., Agoreyo F., Okonofua F. E., "Complete androgen insensitivity syndrome with persistent Mullerian derivatives: a case report." *J Obstet Gynaecol* 2005; 25 (4): 403–5.

[18] Mazur T., "Gender dysphoria and gender change in androgen insensitivity or micropenis." *Arch Sex Behav* 2005;34 (4): 411–21.

[19] Cools M., Drop SLS, Wolff enbuttel K. P., Oosterhuis J. W., Looijenga LHJ. Germ cell tumors in the intersex gonad: old paths, new directions, moving frontiers. *Endocr Rev* 2006; 27: 468–84.

[20] Hughes I. A., Houk C., Ahmed S. F., Lee P. A., "Consensus statement on management of intersex disorders." *Arch. Dis. Child.* 2006; 91 (7): 554–63.

[21] Wooster R., Mangion J., Eeles R., Smith S., Dowsett M., Averill Det al. "A germline mutation in the androgen receptor gene in two brothers with breast cancer and Reifenstein syndrome." *Nat. Genet.* 1992; 2 (2): 132–4.

[22] Lund A., Juvonen V., Lähdetie J., Aittomäki K., Tapanainen J. S., Savontaus M L., "A novel sequence variation in the transactivation regulating domain of the androgen receptor in two infertile Finnish men." *Fertil. Steril.* 1993; 79 Suppl 3: 1647–8.

[23] Lobaccaro J.M., Lumbroso S., Belon C., Galtier-Dereure F., Bringer J., Lesimple T et al. "Androgen receptor gene mutation in male breast cancer." *Hum. Mol. Genet.* 1993; 2 (11): 1799–80.

[24] Enas B. A., Harper M. E., Daniells C. E., Watts C. E., Matenhelia S., Green J., Griffiths K., "Low incidence of androgen receptor gene mutations in human prostatic tumors using single strand conformation polymorphism analysis." *Prostate* 1996; 28 (3): 162–71.

[25] Zuccarello D., Ferlin A., Vinanzi C., et al. Detailed functional studies on androgen receptor mild mutations demonstrate their association with male infertility. *Clin Endocrinol* (Oxf) 2008; 68: 580–88.

[26] La Spada AR, Wilson EM, Lubahn DB, Harding AE, Fischbeck KH. Androgen receptor gene mutations in X-linked spinal and bulbar muscular atrophy. *Nature* 1991; 352: 77–79.

[27] Chang C. S., Kokontis J., Liao S. T., "Molecular cloning of human and rat complementary DNA encoding androgen receptors." *Science* 1988 240 (4850): 324–6.

[28] Trapman J., Klaassen P., Kuiper G. G., van der Korput J. A., Faber P. W., van Rooij H. C., et al. "Cloning, structure and expression of a cDNA encoding the human androgen receptor." *Biochem. Biophys. Res. Commun.* 1988; 153 (1): 241–8.

[29] Roy A. K., Lavrovsky Y., Song C. S., Chen S., Jung M. H., Velu N. K., et al. "Regulation of androgen action." *Vitam. Horm.* 1999; Vitamins and Hormones 55: 309–52.

[30] Rajender S., Singh L., Thangaraj K., "Phenotypic heterogeneity of mutations in androgen receptor gene." *Asian J. Androl.*2007: 9 (2): 147–79.

[31] Matias P. M., Donner P., Coelho R., Thomaz M., Peixoto C., Macedo S., et al. Structural evidence for ligand specificity in the binding domain of the human androgen receptor. Implications for pathogenic gene mutations. *J Biol Chem* 2000; 275: 26164–71.

[32] Koch C. A., Kemp S., Androgen Insensitivity Syndrome. 2004[Online] Available from: http://emedicine.medscape.com/article/924996-overview#a6 Accessed 24th June 2015.

[33] Gottlieb B., Beitel L. K., Trifiro M. A., "Variable expressivity and mutation databases: The androgen receptor gene mutations database." *Hum. Mutat.* 2001 17 (5): 382–8.

[34] Evan B. A. J., Jones T. R., Hughes I. A., Studies of the androgen receptor in dispersed fibroblasts: investigation of patients with androgen insensitivity. *Clin Endocrinol* (Oxf) 1984; 20: 93–105.

[35] Coutant R., Mallet D., Lahlou N., Bouhours-Nouet N., Guichet A., Coupris L., et al. "Heterozygous mutation of steroidogenic factor-1 in 46,XY subjects may mimic partial androgen insensitivity syndrome." *J. Clin. Endocrinol. Metab.* 2007; 92 (8). 2868–73.

[36] Adachi M., Takayanagi R., Tomura A., Imasaki K., Kato S., Goto K., Yanase T., Ikuyama S., Nawata H., (September 2000). "Androgen-insensitivity syndrome as a possible coactivator disease." *N. Engl. J. Med.* 2000; 343 (12): 856–62.

[37] Australian Paediatric Endocrine Group. Submission 88 to the Senate inquiry into the involuntary or coerced sterilization of people with disabilities in Australia: *Regarding the management of children with disorders of sex development.* 2013.

[38] Manuel M., Katayama P. K., Jones H. W., "The age of occurrence of gonadal tumors in intersex patients with a Y chromosome." *Am. J. Obstet. Gynecol.* 1976; 124 (3): 293–300.

[39] Marcus R., Leary D., Schneider D. L., Shane E., Favus M., Quigley C. A., "The contribution of testosterone to skeletal development and maintenance: lessons from the androgen insensitivity syndrome." *J. Clin. Endocrinol. Metab.* 2000; 85 (3): 1032–7.

[40] Soule S. G., Conway G., Prelevic G. M., Prentice M., Ginsburg J., Jacobs H. S., "Osteopenia as a feature of the androgen insensitivity syndrome." *Clin. Endocrinol.* (Oxf) 1995; 43 (6): 671–5.

[41] Ismail-Pratt I. S., Bikoo M., Liao L. M., Conway G. S., Creighton S. M., Normalization of the vagina by dilator treatment alone in Complete Androgen Insensitivity Syndrome and Mayer-Rokitansky-Kuster-Hauser Syndrome. *Hum Reprod* 2007; 22: 2020–24.

[42] Oakes MB, Eyvazzadeh AD, Quint E, Smith YR. "Complete androgen insensitivity syndrome--a review." *J Pediatr Adolesc Gynecol* 2008; 21 (6): 305–10.
[43] Minto C. L., Liao L. M., Woodhouse C. R., Ransley P. G., Creighton S. M., "The effect of clitoral surgery on sexual outcome in individuals who have intersex conditions with ambiguous genitalia: a cross-sectional study." *Lancet* 2003; 361 (9365): 1252–7.
[44] Meyer-Bahlburg H. F., "Gender assignment and reassignment in 46,XY pseudohermaphroditism and related conditions." *J. Clin. Endocrinol. Metab.* 1999; 84 (10): 3455–8.
[45] Danilovic D. L., Correa P. H., Costa E. M., Melo K. F., Mendonca B. B., Arnhold IJ "Height and bone mineral density in androgen insensitivity syndrome with mutations in the androgen receptor gene." *Osteoporos Int* 2007; 18 (3): 369–74.
[46] Ferlin A., Vinanzi C., Garolla A., Selice R., Zuccarello D., Cazzadore C., et al. "Male infertility and androgen receptor gene mutations: clinical features and identification of seven novel mutations." *Clin. Endocrinol.* (Oxf) 2006; 65 (5): 606–10.
[47] Stouffs K., Tournaye H., Liebaers I., Lissens W., "Male infertility and the involvement of the X chromosome." *Hum. Reprod. Update* 2009; 15 (6): 623–37.
[48] Zenteno J. C., Chávez B., Vilchis F., Kofman-Alfaro S., "Phenotypic heterogeneity associated with identical mutations in residue 870 of the androgen receptor." *Horm. Res.* 2002; 57 (3-4): 90–3.
[49] Hiort O., Holterhus P. M., Horter T., Schulze W., Kremke B., Bals-Pratsch M., et al. "Significance of mutations in the androgen receptor gene in males with idiopathic infertility." *J. Clin. Endocrinol. Metab.* 2000; 85 (8): 2810–5.
[50] Dejager S., Bry-Gauillard H., Bruckert E., Eymard B., Salachas F., LeGuern E., et al. "A comprehensive endocrine description of Kennedy's disease revealing androgen insensitivity linked to CAG repeat length." *J. Clin. Endocrinol. Metab.* 2002; 87 (8): 3893–901.
[51] Yong E. L., Ng S. C., Roy A. C., Yun G., Ratnam S. S., "Pregnancy after hormonal correction of severe spermatogenic defect due to mutation in androgen receptor gene." *Lancet* 1994; 344 (8925): 826–7.
[52] Weidemann W., Peters B., Romalo G., Spindler K. D., Schweikert H. U., "Response to androgen treatment in a patient with partial androgen insensitivity and a mutation in the deoxyribonucleic acid-binding domain of the androgen receptor." *J. Clin. Endocrinol. Metab.* 1998; 83 (4): 1173–6.
[53] Nieschlag E., "Testosterone treatment comes of age: new options for hypogonadal men." *Clin. Endocrinol.* (Oxf) 2006; 65 (3): 275–81.

In: Amenorrhea
Editor: Oliver Chukwujekwu Ezechi

ISBN: 978-1-63484-778-0

Chapter 8

GONADAL DYSGENESIS

Cyril C. Dim
Departments of Obstetrics and Gynaecology/Physiology,
Faculty of Medical Sciences, College of Medicine,
University of Nigeria, Enugu, Nigeria

ABSTRACT

Gonadal dysgenesis is a group of disorders that results from chromosomal anomalies and it is usually associated with amenorrhea in affected females. Gonadal dysgenesis can be complete (CGD) or partial (PGD). Within these broad categories, the disorders peculiar to females include monosomy X (45X), Swyer syndrome (46XY CGD), 46XX CGD, and Turner syndrome mosaiscm (45X/XX or XY). Optimal testicular and ovarian differentiation requires Y chromosome with sex-determining region and a complete second X chromosome respectively. Turner syndrome (TS) has typical features and can be diagnosed as early as in prenatal period while 46XX and 46XY CGD may only be obvious during adolescence when the affected individuals fail to enter puberty. Timely replacement of appropriate hormones ensures optimal growth for TS patients as well as the development of secondary sexual characters for all categories of CGD. Conception is only possible in CGD through in vitro fertilization using donor eggs. Cases of gonadal dysgenesis where karyotyping shows presence of Y chromosome will benefit from prophylactic gonadectomy because of risk of malignant transformation.

Keywords: gondal dysgenesis, conception, fertilization, sexual differentiation

INTRODUCTION

Gonadal dysgenesis is a class of disorders of sex development (DSD) characterized by incomplete or defective differentiation of the indifferent embryonic gonads to ovaries or testes due to structural or numerical anomaly of the sex chromosomes. It is a relatively rare compendium of chromosomal disorders that is known to cause amenorrhea in phenotypic females. Depending on the gonadal morphology, gonadal dysgenesis is broadly classified into complete or partial; the latter is also referred to as mixed gonadal dysgenesis. In the complete type (CGD) such as 46XY (Swyer syndrome) and 45X (Turner syndrome), there is no gonadal development thus the affected individual has a complete female phenotype while in the partial type (PGD), X and Y chromosomes may coexist leading to the development of ovary and/or testes thus the external genitalia will depend on the degree of functionality of the testis. For example, in Turner mosaic 45X/46XX, the individual is phenotypically female while mosaic 45X/46XY may have incomplete genital masculization. The problem in this group of diseases is primarily at the level of gonads and they are therefore part of the entity referred to as primary gonadal disorders with hormonal pattern of hypergonadotropic hypogonadism. Because of the arrest of development of the indifferent gonads and absence of germ cells histologically in CGD especially, the gonads consist of fibrous tissue and are known as streak gonads. Gonadal dysgenesis affect both males and females however, since this book is dedicated to oligomenorhea/amenorrhrea, further discussions in this chapter are restricted to the categories of gonadal dysgenesis that have female phenotype.

PATHOGENESIS

Sexual differentiation of the genital system appears to be sequential thus: differentiation from genetic sex to gonadal sex to ductal sex, and finally to genital sex. Humans are made up of both somatic (diploid) and germ cells (haploid). The former consist of 44 pairs of autosomal chromosomes and two sex chromosomes. The genetic sex is determined by the sex chromosomes thus a pair of X chromosomes in females, and a combination of X and Y chromosomes in males. The genetic composition of female germ cell (ovum) is 23X while that of males (spermatozoa) can be 23X or 23Y. When an X chromosome bearing spermatozoa fertilizes an ovum, a genetic female is formed but, when Y containing spermatozoa fertilizes an ovum, genetic male forms. Furthermore, in the presence of a Y chromosome bearing the sex determining gene, testes are formed otherwise the ovaries develop. The sex determining gene, located in the sex- determining region of Y chromosomes (SRY), is responsible for initiating the transcription of genes necessary for testicular differentiation and production of mullerian inhibiting substance (MIS). The latter is a glycoprotein produced by the fetal testis and it acts locally (paracrine function) to cause the regression of the mullerian duct thereby preventing the development of fallopian tubes, uterus, and upper vagina. Therefore, the Y-chromosome is necessary for development of a genetic male and testes (gonadal male). On the other hand, when the Y chromosome is absent (e.g., 45X Turner syndrome) or defective (e.g., 46XY, Swyer syndrome), the testes will not develop and the MIS and testosterone will not be produced so, the internal and external genitalia will remain female. In other words, default setting for the development of the genital system is female (Figure 1) unless directed by male factors thus: Y-chromosome (with sex-determining region) and testis. Furthermore, it is believed that a complete development of the ovaries requires two X-chromosomes which may explain why an X monosomy female develops premature degeneration of germ cells and has no ovarian follicles - ovarian follicles do not appear in the absence of oocytes.

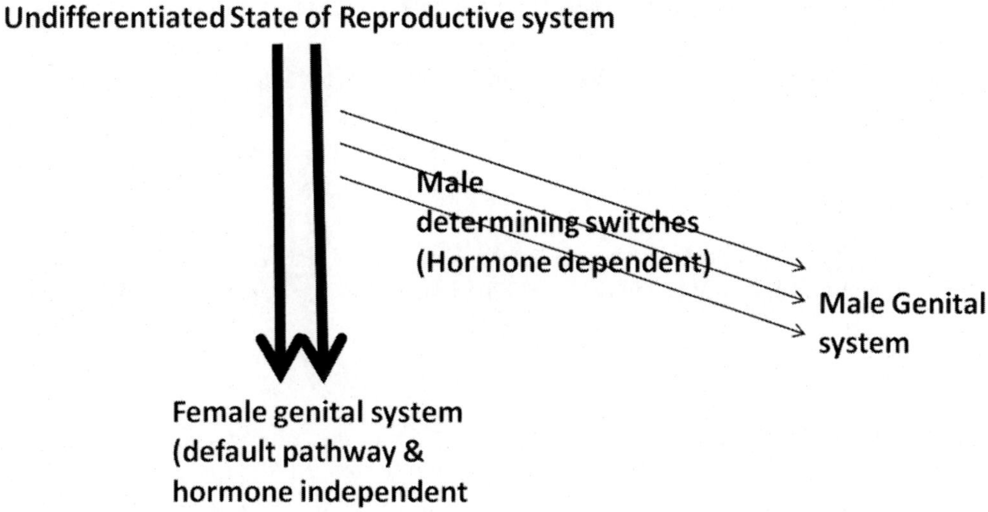

Figure 1. Default setting for development of human reproductive system.

Complete Gonadal Dysgenesis

In this group of disorders, differentiated gonads are absent, but the female internal and external genitalia develop. The karyotype is usually 45X, 46XY or 46XX.

The 45X complete gonadal dysgenesis otherwise called classical Turner syndrome or monosomy X constitutes about 50% of Turner syndrome (TS) – an entity that was first described by Henry Turner in 1938. Generally, in this syndrome, one or part of the second X chromosome in some or all cells of a female is missing. It is the commonest form of gonadal dysgenesis with an incidence of up to 1 in 2000 live-born female infants. There is neither racial/ethnic predisposition nor relationship with maternal age. 45X CGD is a common chromosomal abnormality in spontaneous abortuses - it constituted 16.5% of all spontaneous abortus cases in a Turkish population. Generally, it is the absence of one set of genes from the short arm of one X chromosome that causes Turner syndrome. However, in 45X CGD, there is post-zygotic loss of the second sex chromosome (monosomy) early in embryonic life, and most of the lost chromosomes are usually paternal in origin. Also, affected individual may have partial monosomy such as a deletion of the short arm of one of the two X chromosomes or the presence of an isochromosome with two long arms.

Table 1. Definitions of common gene symbols implicated in female gonadal dysgenesis

Gene symbol	Protein name	Chromosomal locus
SRY	Sex-determining region Y or testis determining factor	Yp11.3
DHH	Desert hedgehog	12q13.1
MAP3K1	Mitogen-activated protein kinase kinase kinase 1	5q11.2
NR5A1	Nuclear receptor subfamily 5, group A, member 1	9q33
FSHR	follicle stimulating hormone receptor	2p21-p16
BMP15	bone morphogenetic protein 15	Xp11.2
SHOX	Short stature homeobox	Xp22.33

The 46XY complete gonadal dysgenesis (46XY CGD) was first described by G. J. Swyer and is often referred to as Swyer syndrome. It has a prevalence of approximately 1 in 80,000 individuals. In this condition, the Y chromosome of the affected individual lacks the capacity to switch on testicular development and embryonic function so, the female internal and external genitalia develop. In a majority of affected patients, the aetiology is a mutation of the SRY gene or other genes associated with sexual differentiation including *DHH*, *MAP3K1*, *NR5A1* genes (Table 1).

For the 46XX CGD, prevalence is less than 1 per 10,000 individuals. In most cases, the aetiology is unknown, however, inheritable mutations of several genes have been implicated including *FSHR, BMP15, NR5A1* genes (Table 1).

Partial Gonadal Dysgenesis

Partial gonadal dysgenesis (PGD) is a group of diseases that are caused by chromosomal mosaicism. The PGD of interest in this discussion is Turner mosaicism (45X/46XX or XY). In this case, there are two cell lines with 45X chromosomal abnormality present in one of the cell lines while the other cell line usually carries 46XX, or occasionally 46XY. In the latter, the proportion of Y chromosome material is not adequate to initiate the development of male features, but is associated with an increased risk of malignant transformation of the gonads. As a rule, the phenotype of the affected individual must be female for this diagnosis (TS) to be made. Turner mosaicism constitutes about 30% of TS cases.

Clinical Features

All categories of gonadal dysgenesis have one common feature which is female phenotype. Also, a majority of them have primary or secondary amenorrhea.

Adults with CGD (45X and 46XY or XX CGD) have streaked gonads, primary amenorrhea with elevated luteinizing hormone (LH) and follicule stimulating hormone (FSH), as well as absent secondary sexual characteristics including breast development. In addition 45X CGD have short stature due to slower growth rate in childhood and absent growth spurt in adolescence. It is believed that the loss of one *SHOX* gene on the affected X chromosome is responsible for the short stature. 45X CGD also express various combinations of the features of Turner syndrome such as a high arched palate with or without dental crowding, webbed neck, cubitus valgus (wide carrying angle), normal pubic hairs, broad chest and widely spaced nipples, short fourth metacarpal or metatarsal, hypoplastic or hyperconvex nails, excessive nevi when compared to siblings, cardiovascular malformations include hypoplastic left heart and aortic dissection, otitis media, and thyroid dysfunction. TS females have normal intelligence though some learning disabilities may occur. The X chromosomes contain many important genes including genes for ovarian development, height, sexual development etc, which explains the range of clinical presentations of the TS.

Unlike TS females, individuals with 46XY or XX CGD usually do not have obvious abnormalities and are often only detected when menarche does not occur or secondary sex characteristics fail to develop during adolescence. For individual with 46XY CCD, the associated dysgenetic gonads have potential for malignant transformation to dysgerminoma, gonadoblastoma, etc which can occur as early as age of ten years.

Turner mosaicism has varying somatic abnormalities but it is still classified as turner syndrome from a genetic point of view. Therefore, individuals with Turner mosaicism have characteristic feature of short stature and may have other combinations of TS features. Depending on the proportion of 45X cells, some of the affected females may develop secondary sexual characteristics and a small proportion of this group can conceive spontaneously though they have higher risk of premature ovarian failure later in adult life. Like in Sweyer syndrome, very small proportion of Turner mosaicism, where one of the cell lines contains Y chromosome, has higher risk of malignant transformation of the gonads.

DIAGNOSIS AND TREATMENT

For TS to be diagnosed, the affected individual must be female in the presence of the typical phenotypic features as well as a standard 30-cell karyotype analysis that shows a complete (monosomy X) or partial absence of a second sex chromosome (TS mosaicism). It is important to investigate affected females for the presence of Y chromosomal material because of the associated risk of malignancy. Fetal ultrasonography may suggest TS when nuchal cystic hygroma, horseshoe kidney, left-sided cardiac anomalies, or nonimmune fetal hydrops are observed. Prenatal diagnoses are confirmed by amniocentesis or chorionic villous sampling karyotyping.

TS is a lifelong condition that has no cure but there are multi-disciplinary treatments that can alleviate the impacts of its symptoms. The concern of this section is in the treatment of menstrual and reproduction related features of the condition. Growth hormone therapy started early in life and stopped at onset of puberty will improve the height of affected girls when diagnosed early in life. Also, it has been suggested that combining growth hormone with ultra-low-dose estrogen in childhood may improve the growth of affected females. Furthermore, estrogen and progesterone therapy introduced at about age of 12 years will initiate puberty and associated development of secondary sexual characteristics. The above hormone treatments will not improve the fertility potentials of the affected individuals, therefore, those desirous of conception will benefit from in vitro fertilization and embryo transfer (IVF-ET) using donor eggs. Turner mosaic girls with Y chromosomes in one of their cell lines should have surgical removal of the dysgenetic gonads as soon as possible because of the increased risk of malignant transformation.

For 46XY or XX CGD, diagnosis usually occurs at puberty when primary amenorrhea develops because of lack of major ovarian steroids. The affected individual should have both female internal and external genitalia with undeveloped streaked gonads lacking germ cells, as well a cell karyotype of 46XY (Sweyer syndrome) or 46XX. Typical features of TS including short stature are absent. There is normal hypothalamic-pituitary axis with features of hypergonadotropic hypogonadism. As in classical TS, estrogen and progesterone therapy leads to normal puberty. Also, conception is only possible through IVF-ET with donor egg. Most importantly, prophylactic gonadectomy is indicated in 46XY CGD for reasons already discussed; annual abdominal sonograms are recommended to evaluate for malignant changes till the surgery is carried out. Genetic counseling and evaluation of at-risk relatives are indicated because of possible hereditary nature of the condition.

Conclusion

Gonadal dysgenesis is broadly classified into complete and partial with varying prevalence. The categories of gonadal dysgenesis with female internal and external genitalia include classical TS or monosomy X (45X), Sweyer syndrome (46XY), 46XX CGD, and TS mosaiscm (45X/XX or XY). Y chromosome with functional SRY is required for optimal testicular differentiation and functions. Also, a complete second X chromosome is necessary for the development of ovaries. TS usually have characteristic features and can be diagnosed prenatally or during childhood while 46XX or XY CGD may only be obvious when primary amenorrhea develops during adolescence. Appropriate hormone replacement ensures optimal growth for TS patients as well as the development of secondary sexual characters for all cases of CGD. Conception is achievable in CGD through IVF-ET using donor eggs. Swyer syndrome and 46XX CGD have hereditary potentials so, genetic counseling should be part of the management of affected individuals. Prophylactic gonadectomy is recommended for cases of gonadal dysgenesis with Y chromosome because of risk of malignant transformation. Finally, gonadal dysgenesis affects reproductive development in females therefore, early diagnoses and timely initiation of treatment are necessary to improve reproductive functions.

References

Alpman A, Cogulu O, Akgul M, et al. Prenatally Diagnosed Turner Syndrome and Cystic Hygroma: Incidence and Reasons for Referrals. *Fetal Diagn Ther.* 2008; 25: 58-61.

Baronchelli S, Conconi D, Panzeri E, et al. Cytogenetics of premature ovarian failure: an investigation on 269 affected women. *J Biomed Biotechnol.* 2011; 2011:370195.

Bauman D. Pediatric and Adolescent Gynecology. In: DeCherney AH, Nathan L, Laufer N, Roman AS, editors. Current Obstetrics and Gynecologic Diagnosis and Treatment 11th ed. New York: *McGraw-Hill* 2013. p. 582 – 610.

Carr RF, Ochs RH, Ritter DA, Kenny JD, Fridey JL, Ming PM. Fetal cystic hygroma and Turner's syndrome. *Am J Dis Child.* 1986; 140: 580-3.

Crespi B. Turner syndrome and the evolution of human sexual dimorphism. *Evol Appl* 2008; 1: 449–61.

Cunningham FG, Leveno KJ, Bloom SL, Hauth JC, Rouse DJ, Spong CY. Williams Obstetrics 23rd ed. USA: McGraw-Hill 2010 p. 103.

Daniel MS, Postellon DC. Turner Syndrome. Available at: http://emedicine.medscape.com/article/949681-overview. Accessed on 10 June 2015.

Davenport ML. Approach to the patient with Turner syndrome. *J Clin Endocrinol Metab.* 2010 95: 1487-95.

Donaldson MD, Gault EJ, Tan KW, Dunger DB. Optimising management in Turner syndrome: from infancy to adult transfer. Arch Dis Child. 2006 91: 513-20.

Gene Review. Available at: http://www.ncbi.nlm.nih.gov/books/NBK1547/. Accessed on 17 June 2015.

Genetic Home Reference. Swyer syndrome. Available at: http://ghr.nlm.nih. gov/condition/swyer-syndrome. Accessed on 17 June 2015.

HUGO Gene Nomenclature Committee. Available at: http://www.genenames.org/Accessed on: 5 July 2015.

Hughes IA, Houk C, Ahmed SF, Lee PA; LWPES Consensus Group; ESPE Consensus Group. Consensus statement on management of intersex disorders. *Arch Dis Child* 2006; 91: 554–63.

Hughes IA. Disorders of sex development: a new definition and classification. *Best Pract Res Clin Endocrinol Metab* 2008; 22: 119–34.

Hutcheson J, Snyder III HM. Disorders of Sexual Development Follow-up. Available at: http://emedicine.medscape.com/article/1015520. Accessed on 2 July 2015.

Leigh B, Dorn C, Ulrich U. Gonadal dysgenesis. *Gynakol Geburtsmed Gynakol Endokrinol* 2009; 5: 82–94.

MacLaughlin DT, Donahoe PK. Sex determination and differentiation. *N Engl J Med.* 2004 22; 350: 367-78.

McCann-Crosby B, Mansouri R, Dietrich JE, et al. State of the art review in gonadal dysgenesis: challenges in diagnosis and management. *Int J Pediatr Endocrinol.* 2014; 2014: 4.

Michala L, Goswami D, Creighton SM, Conway GS. Swyer syndrome: presentation and outcomes. *BJOG* 2008; 115: 737–41.

National organization for Rare Disorders (NORD). Turner Syndrome. Available at: https://rarediseases.org/rare-diseases/turner-syndrome/. Accessed On: July 5, 2015.

Orphanet. 46,XX gonadal dysgenesis. Available at: http://www.orpha.net/consor/cgi-bin/OC_Exp.php?lng=EN&Expert=243. Accessed on 10 June 2015.

Ostrer H. 46,XY Disorder of Sex Development and 46,XY Complete Gonadal Dysgenesis.

Ostrer H. Disorders of Sex Development (DSDs): An Update. *J Clin Endocrinol Metab* 2014; 99: 1503 – 09.

Ross JL, Quigley CA, Cao D, et al. Growth hormone plus childhood low-dose estrogen in Turner's syndrome. *N Engl J Med.* 2011; 364: 1230-42.

Shahid M, Dhillon VS, Hussain Z, et al. Analysis of the SRY gene in two sex-reversed XY sisters identifies two new novel point mutations in the high mobility group box domain. *Fertil Steril* 2008; 90: 1199.e1–8.

Swyer GIM. Male pseudohermaphroditism: a hitherto undecribed form. *Br Med J* 1955; 2: 707-12.

Turner HH. A syndrome of infantilism, congenital webbed neck, and cubitus valgus. *Endocrinology* 1938; 23: 566–74.

Yakut S, Toru HS, Cetin Z, et al. Chromosome abnormalities identified in 457 spontaneous abortions and their histopathological findings. *Turk Patoloji Derg.* 2015; 31: 111-8.

In: Amenorrhea
Editor: Oliver Chukwujekwu Ezechi

ISBN: 978-1-63484-778-0

Chapter 9

CRYPTOMENORRHEA

Carol Odula[1] and Oliver Chukwujekwu Ezechi[2]
[1]University of Nairobi Health Services, Nairobi, Kenya
[2]Clinical Sciences Division, Nigerian Institute of Medical Research, Lagos, Nigeria

ABSTRACT

Obstruction of the lower genital tract leading to amenorrhea is uncommon However, knowledge of the clinical presentation and management of these cases is central in order to avoid sequel consequent on misdiagnosis or mismanagement. Cryptomenorrhoea may be caused by an isolated congenital abnormalities, trauma or infection of the lower genital tract. Occasionally, congenital causes may be associated with more complex syndromes, and the importance of these relationships needs to be understood by those managing gynaecological issues of women. Cultural, psychological, medical and surgical issues often arose in the management of patient with this condition. The best patient outcome requires a multidisciplinary team approach.

Keywords: cryptomenorrhoea, amenorrhea, haematocolpos, haematometra

INTRODUCTION

The patent genital tract is important for the expulsion of cervical and vaginal secretion, as well as the efflux of the menstruum [1]. Cryptomenorrhea or retained menstruation amenorrhea occurs when the menstrual blood is unable to flow out due to an obstruction in the tract in a woman that has normal periods. The obstruction may occur at different levels with resultant variations in clinical presentation. In hematocolpos, the accumulation of menstrual blood in the vagina and hematometra when there is accumulation of menstrual blood in the uterus. Often there is associated monthly period pain or other menstrual symptoms.

EPIDEMIOLOGY

The malformations of the female genital tract rare and are usually accompanied by other abnormalities, especially related to the kidneys, urinary tract, and bones. It is estimated that about 33% of such malformations are associated with other anomalies. Imperforate hymen is the most common genital outflow tract anomaly. Müllerian agenesis is rare and occurs in about one in 4000 - 5000 women [1, 2].

PATHOGENESIS

The urogenital system develops from the intermediate mesothelium of the peritoneal cavity and the endoderm of the urogenital sinus. The presence of a Y chromosome leads to male sex determination and in its absence and in the presence of two X chromosomes, the Wolffian ducts regress due to a lack of testosterone and the Müllerian ducts persist due to the absence of Müllerian inhibitory factor. The lower two thirds of the vagina develop from the urogenital sinus, while the upper vagina, cervix, uterus, fallopian tubes, and ovaries develop from the Müllerian duct system. Failure of vertical fusion or canalization of the two systems in utero may result in cervical stenosis or atresia, vaginal atresia, transverse vaginal septum, and imperforate hymen. Obstruction may also occur along the lower genital tract as a result of stenosis of the cervix or atresia of the vagina [1, 2]. Irrespective of the mechanism of occurrence, though the endometrium is shed cyclically, the obstruction retains the menstrual flow causing accumulation of blood in the vagina (hematocolpos) or uterus (hematometra) depending on the level of the obstruction. In neglected cases, the blood may enter the fallopian tubes and endometrium with formation of adhesion and haematosalpinx.

AETIOLOGY AND CLASSIFICATION

Defect in the normal organogenesis involving the urogenital sinus, the Müllerian duct or trauma during cervical surgery or neglected difficulty vaginal delivery can result in stenosis, atresia or obstruction of the lower genital tract. Recent interest on the abnormalities in the structure; expression or function of the mammalian *HOX* genes has led insinuations that it may be a possible cause of the congenital malformations of the lower genital tract [2, 3]. Other causes of outflow obstructions include scarring of the vagina and vaginal agglutination as result of infection or insertion of corrosive in the vagina. (Table 1)

CLINICAL FEATURES

Most patients with outflow tract obstruction present with a history of amenorrhea, recurrent cyclical lower abdominal discomfort or pain, or lower abdominal midline mass. In long standing cases the patient may present with symptoms of complications of haematocolpos, haematometra or haematoslpix such as urinary retention, constipation, and hydronephrosis (Table 2). In case of imperforate hymen patient complain of a mass in the vagina.

Physical examination findings may depend on the level of the obstruction. In cases due to imperforation of hymen, the hymen may bulge and exhibit a bluish discoloration. In cases of transverse vaginal septum, physical findings depend on the site and level of the septum. A bulging septum may be felt during pelvic examination reveal the presence of the. In addition the vagina is short and observed as a blind pouch. A uniform and global mid line lower abdominal mass could be seen or palpable in long standing cases with haematometra.

Table 1. Classification and causes of Cryptomenorrhea

A. Aetiology
    1. Congenital
        i. Imperforate hymen
        ii. Transverse vaginal septum
        iii. Atresia of upper vagina and or cervix
        iv. Congenital absence of the vagina with intact uterus
    2. Acquired
        i. Trauma
            1. Cervical stenosis due to conisation or cauterisation
            2. Vaginal atresia
                a. Difficult and neglected vaginal delivery
                b. Insertion of corrosive chemicals
            3. Labial agglutination from genital mutilation
        ii. Infection
            1. Lichen planus infection of the vagina
        iii. Radiation therapy
            1. Management of genital cancers e.g., cervix, endometrial

B. Presentation
    1. Haematocolpos
    2. Haemometra
    3. Haematosalpinx

Table 2. Potential complications of outflow obstruction of lower genital tract

1. Hematocolpos
2. Hematometra
3. Pyohematocolpos
4. Pyohematometra
5. Urinary retention, hydronephrosis (rare)
6. Postoperative recurrence of obstruction
7. Constipation
8. Abdominal mass

DIFFERENTIAL DIAGNOSIS

Other condition to be considered in a patient present with amenorrhea, and or abdominal are listed in the Table 3.

Table 3. Differential diagnosis of amenorrhea due to outflow tract abnormality

Clinical Condition	Differentiating feature
Vaginal cyst	No amenorrhea
Vaginal tumours	No amenorrhea Presence of constitutional symptoms in malignant cases
Müllerian agenesis	No cyclical abdominal pain or abdominal mass
Androgen Insensitivity syndrome	No cyclical abdominal pain or abdominal mass Scanty or absent axillary and public hair

MANAGEMENT

Diagnosis of amenorrhea due to cryptomenorrhoea could be made in majority of cases after a detailed history and physical examination. In some situation further investigation may be necessary to confirm the diagnosis.

Failure to menstruation in teenage and adult women generates understandable anxiety with regard to sexuality, sexual function and reproduction. The issues are complex psychologically, culturally as well as gynaecological. Multidimensional nature of issues involved in this condition illustrates superior outcome for patients treated by a multidisciplinary team.

Diagnosis

In situation where history and physical examination could not confirm the diagnosis, examination under anaesthesia will be required. Under anaesthesia, vaginoscopy or direct inspection of the vagina with a nasal speculum and a light source should be performed. Documentation of the findings should be meticulous and photographs taken only with appropriate consent [2, 4].

Trans-abdominal ultrasound assessment of the pelvis is invaluable when bimanual examination is inappropriate and/or there is reason to question internal organ development and potential functional integrity [4, 5]. Three-dimensional ultrasound scan of the pelvis can reveal additional associated congenital malformations of the uterus or cervix. It also reveals hematocolpos or hematometra. Magnetic resonance imaging can delineate other associated abnormalities of the urinary tract. An accurate and full assessment of the underlying anatomy is important for patients undergoing surgery, before the operation is performed.

Fluid culture is helpful in determining appropriate antibiotic therapy, in rare cases of transverse vaginal septum, in which ascending infection as result of previous mismanagement may lead to pyohematometra.

Karyotyping or serum testosterone levels are required to exclude the diagnosis of androgen insensitivity syndrome in patients with blind vaginal pouch and scanty pubic or axillary hair.

Treatment

Counselling

Adequate counselling of the patients and their family is necessary before any treatment as this is as important as the treatment itself. Cultural considerations regarding the importance of a certain appearance of the hymen, as an indication of virginity, and the meaning of the term virginity, should be discussed before surgery. Surgical correction of the obstruction is a medical necessity. Cultural views, while respected, should not preclude the performance of an appropriate surgical procedure [6-8]. Counselling should include detail information about the possible aetiology. In acquired causes of cryptomenorrhoea, patient should be educated in dangers of applying unapproved chemicals into the vagina for any reason.

Surgical Management

1. Imperforate Hymen

Oral contraceptive to suppress menses allows symptomatic relief and time required to complete further investigation. Nonsteroidal anti-inflammatory drugs can be given to provide pain relief. Narcotic analgesics are really required.

The appropriate time to operate an imperforate hymen is based on the presence and severity of symptoms. A symptomatic mucocele presenting in the neonatal period should be treated expediently but is not considered a surgical emergency [5, 7]. Asymptomatic imperforate hymen without a mucocele during childhood, should be delayed to the onset of puberty and prior to the development of a hematocolpos or hematometra. The presence of estrogen stimulation in puberty facilitates surgical repair and healing. While expedient treatment of an imperforate hymen is appropriate when it manifests in an adolescent with hematometra and hematocolpos, the procedure should not be performed on an emergent basis without an appropriate preoperative evaluation. Aspiration or puncture of the mucocolpos or hematocolpos without definitive enlargement of the vaginal orifice should be avoided because a pyocolpos or ascending infection may develop, setting the stage for pyocolpos or pyometrium, with the potential to adversely affect fertility [2, 5].

The aim of a hymenotomy procedure is to open the hymenal membrane in such a way as to leave a normally patent vaginal orifice that does not scar [5]. Pre-emptive analgesia is important. This involves the infiltration of the membrane prior to the incision with a long-acting local anesthetic (e.g., 0.25% bupivacaine). Large hematocolpos are typically under pressure, and the surgeon should be prepared to evacuate the content using suction cannulae. The initial incision in the hymenal membrane could be revised only after the evacuation of the hematocolpos. A cruciate incision along the diagonal diameters of the hymen, rather than anterior to posterior is advocated as it avoids injury to the urethra and can be enlarged by removal of excess hymenal tissue. Alternatively the hymenal orifice is enlarged using a circular incision following the lines of the normal annular hymenal configuration [5-8]. Occasional significant bleeding requires using interrupted stitches with fine absorbable suture to achieve haemostasis. Postoperative analgesia should be provided with the application of 2% lidocaine jelly to the vaginal introitus. A running interlocking suture is discouraged to minimize circumferential scarring. Relaxing incisions (a radial incision in the hymen that is closed horizontally) may be helpful for ensuring adequate vaginal diameter and minimizing the need for a repeat procedure due to scarring [5].

2. Transverse Vaginal Septum

Transverse vaginal septum commonly occurs between the upper one-third and lower two-thirds of the vaginal canal. The surgery is performed to remove the transverse vaginal septum without significantly shortening the vaginal canal. Operation for a transverse vaginal septum depends on the location, thickness, and need for vaginoplasty. The procedure of choice is incision and drainage of the hematometra or hematocolpos, with reconstruction delayed 6-8 weeks until the tissues have completely healed [9]. Definitive surgery involves the excision of the septum with end-to-end anastomosis of the vaginal walls. Hysteroscopic resection and excision and insertion of a coated tracheobronchial stent to maintain patency until full epithelialization and image-guided balloon vaginoplasty can also be used when available [10-12].

3. Müllerian Agenesis

Vaginal reconstruction should be performed, however, repeat operations are often required, and complications (e.g., stenosis and fistula formation) are not uncommon. Vaginal strictures may also follow, necessitating repeated dilatation [12].

4. Labial Adhesion

Spontaneous resolution has been reported in as many as 80% of non traumatic labial adhesion within 1 year and should be observed. This type of labial adhesions should be managed with periodic observation. Topical estrogen cream is indicated. If treatment in symptomatic or in cases of complete blockage of the vaginal opening, Failure of separation of the labia minora with medical therapy, warrants the consideration of manual or surgical separation. Other reasons to consider intervention include severe fibrous dense adhesions or rare cases with urinary retention [13]. In patient with labial adhesions from lichen sclerosus sharp dissection should be performed separate the adherent labia. Surgicel, oxidized regenerated cellulose gauze should be used to exposed the clitoral hood and labial surfaces with vicryl suture. Complete dissolution of the surgicel is expected 4–6 without recurrence of adhesions [14].

5. Vaginal Atresia or Agenesis

Reconstruction of the vagina is the standard treatment for vaginal atresia, stenosis or agenesis. The ideal neovaginal procedure should provide a patent vaginal canal of adequate length, width, and texture that will allow for sexual intercourse, provide a cosmetically appealing appearance with minimal morbidity of both the recipient and donor surgical sites, and have a low incidence of overall complications [16, 17, 19].

The multiple reconstructive options available for vaginal reconstruction show that no single technique has gained uniform approval. A multidisciplinary approach is recommended to best meet the challenge of providing good cosmetic results with optimal functional and reproductive outcomes [17, 19].

There is no universally acceptable standard procedure for vaginal reconstructive surgery, among a number of surgical and nonsurgical techniques used to create the vagina. The available techniques include vaginal dilation methods, the McIndoe vaginoplasty, modified McIndoe procedures, transpositional skin graft techniques, laparoscopic techniques, myocutaneous and fasciocutaneous pedicled flap surgeries, and intestinal flap surgeries. Each method of repair has its advantages and disadvantages, which should be carefully weighed with the desired treatment goals as well as the surgeon's experience [19].

Surgical approaches for the reconstruction of the vagina can be classified according to the tissues used to create a neovagina (Table 4). Reconstruction involves the use of extra-abdominal tissues or tissues from the abdominal cavity.

Table 4. Surgical approaches for the construction of vagina

Surgical approach	**Tissue used for creating of Neovagina**	**Pros and cons**
A. Vaginal Diltation	No tissue used	Simple, low cost and morbidity, however achieving adequate vaginal depth is a challenge
B. Balloon vaginoplasty	No tissue used	Technically simple, physically safe, and medically effective
C. McIndoe Technique.	Split-thickness skin graft from the buttock	Low morbidity and mortality Tendency to develop vaginal stenosis, lack of natural lubrication, the possible development of fistulas and the need for continuous mold placement if the vagina is not used.
D. Wang Procedure [18]	Musculocutaneous flaps (Rectus and gracilis muscles).	Provide a sensate surface but they are bulky.
E. Lin Procedure	Buccal mucosa	Biological and healing qualities of the buccal mucosa tissue, minimal scarring, and excellent post-operative recovery. Limited vaginal dimensions, and the possibility of either intraoral damage, during tissue-harvesting.
F. Colovaginoplasty	Sigmoid colon along with its vascular pedicle	Potential complications (e.g., diversion colitis) Gives good space and length to neo-vagina.

Table 4. (Continued)

Surgical approach	Tissue used for creating Neovagina	Pros and cons
G. Labia minora flap (Don Flap)	Labia minora	Simple surgical procedure, Need for restorative labiaplasty and cervical dilation to produce an adequate vagina
H. Vecchietti vaginoplasty	Vaginal skin	Vecchietti technique have the highest success rates both anatomically and functionally among available treatments options for vaginal hypoplasia
I. Laparoscopic peritoneal pull through vaginoplasty	Peritoneum	Neovagina has an acidic pH and normal cytology. Low morbidity. Adequate vaginal length and size Offers patients good coital function with natural lubrication and pleasure.

Conclusion

Amenorrhea due to lower genital tract obstruction is rare. Obstetricians and Gynaecologists must be aware of them as they can affect women psychological well-being and fertility if the diagnosis is delayed or mismanaged. Simple obstructive outflow tract disorders, such as an imperforate hymen and thin low transverse septum of the vaginal and labial agglutination can be treated very effectively by the general Gynaecologist but more complex obstructive disorders need the approach of specialist gynaecologic surgeon to obtain optimum results. Pre-operative counselling of patients and their families is as important as the definitive surgery.

References

[1] Dietrich JE, Millar DM, Quint EH. Obstructive reproductive tract anomalies. *J Pediatr Adolesc Gynecol*. 2014 Dec. 27 (6):396-402.

[2] Fotopoulou, Christina, Nicole Gehrmann, Jalid Sehouli, and Werner Lichtenegger. "Reconstructive surgical management of cryptomenorrhea because of complex uterovaginal malformations with duplicate uterus and complete vaginal agenesis." *Fertility and sterility* 2010; 94(6): 2329-e13.

[3] Steinmetz GP. Formation of artificial vagina. *West J Surg* 1940;48:169–3.

[4] Hayden, Catherine J., and Adam H. Balen. "Primary amenorrhea: investigation and treatment." *Obstetrics, Gynaecology and Reproductive Medicine* 2007;17(7): 199-204.

[5] Hillard, P., and J. Adams. "Imperforate hymen." *2012-03-261] http://www. emedicine, conr/med/topic 3329, htm* (2005).

[6] Basaran M, Usal D, Aydemir C. Hymen sparing surgery for imperforate hymen: case reports and review of literature. *J Pediatr Adolesc Gynecol.* 2009;22(4):e61-4.

[7] Dane C, Dane B, Erginbas M, Cetin A. Imperforate hymen-a rare cause of abdominal pain: two cases and review of the literature. *J Pediatr Adolesc Gynecol.* 2007; 20(4):245-7.

[8] Acar A, Balci O, Karatayli R, Capar M, Colakoglu MC. The treatment of 65 women with imperforate hymen by a central incision and application of Foley catheter. *BJOG.* 2007, 114(11):1376-9.

[9] Wheeless, Clifford R. *Atlas of pelvic surgery.* Lippincott Williams and Wilkins, 1997.

[10] Kansagra AP, Miller CB, Roberts AC. A novel image-guided balloon vaginoplasty method to treat obstructive vaginal anomalies. *J Vasc Interv Radiol.* 2011; 22(5):691-4.

[11] Cetinkaya SE, Kahraman K, Sonmezer M, Atabekoglu C. Hysteroscopic management of vaginal septum in a virginal patient with uterus didelphys and obstructed hemivagina. *Fertility and Sterility.* 2011;96:e16-e18.

[12] Cooper AR, Merritt DF. Novel use of a tracheobronchial stent in a patient with uterine didelphys and obstructed hemivagina. *Fertil Steril.* 2010; 93(3):900-3.

[13] Davies MC, Creighton SM, Woodhouse CR. The pitfalls of vaginal construction. *BJU Int.* 2005;95(9):1293-8.

[14] Omar, Hatim A. "Management of labial adhesions in prepubertal girls." *Journal of pediatric and adolescent gynecology* 2000; 13.4: 183-185.

[15] Breech, Lesley L., and Marc R. Laufer. "Surgicel® in the management of labial and clitoral hood adhesions in adolescents with lichen sclerosus." *Journal of pediatric and adolescent gynecology* 2002, 13.1: 21-22.

[16] Edmonds, D. Keith, and Gillian L. Rose. Outflow tract disorders of the female genital tract. *The Obstetrician and Gynaecologist* 2013;15(1): 11-17.

[17] Saxena AK, Paton EA, Windle ML, Wolfram W, Zuckerman AL. Vaginal Atresia Treatment and Management. http://emedicine.medscape. com/article/954110-overview.

[18] Wang X, Qiao Q, Burd A, et al. A new technique of vaginal reconstruction with the deep inferior epigastric perforator flap: a preliminary report. *Plast Reconstr Surg.* 2007; 119(6):1785-90; discussion 1791.

[19] Unger CA, Paraiso MFR. Construction of the Neovagina. In Firoozi F (ed) Female Pelvic Surgery. Springer New York 2015. DOI 10.1007/978-1-4939-1504-0_18.

In: Amenorrhea
Editor: Oliver Chukwujekwu Ezechi

ISBN: 978-1-63484-778-0

Chapter 10

KALLMANN'S SYNDROME

Leonard Ogbonna Ajah[1] and Oliver Chukwujekwu Ezechi[2]
[1]Department of Obstetrics and Gynaecology,
University of Nigeria, Enugu Campus, Enugu, Nigeria
[2]Division of Clinical Sciences,
Nigerian Institute of Medical Research, Lagos, Nigeria

ABSTRACT

Kallmann syndrome (KS) is a genetic disorder characterized by the association of congenital hypogonadotropic hypogonadism and a total or partial lack of sense of smell. KS is due to the deficiency of gonadotropin-releasing hormone (GnRH), with hypoplasia or aplasia of the olfactory bulbs. Though KS occurs in both male and female, it is commoner in males. An estimated prevalence of 1/8,000 males and 1/40,000 females is reported, but is probably underestimated. KS presents with both reproductive and non-reproductive symptoms. Not all symptoms will appear in every case of KS/HH, not even amongst family members. KS is a congenital condition, and therefore exists from birth. However, the genetic basis of these conditions is not fully understood. KS can be inherited through generations, but it is sometimes difficult to predict if this will occur. The diagnosis is often one of exclusion found during the evaluation of a delayed puberty. Differential diagnosis include other forms of hypogonadotrophic hypogonadism and a normal constitutional delay of puberty. The main laboratory findings include low serum testosterone and low levels of the LH and FSH in men, and low serum oestrogen and low levels of LH and FSH in women. Hormonal replacement therapy is used to induce puberty, and later, fertility. There is currently no treatment for anosmia. KS is not a life threatening condition. With hormonal treatment, puberty occurs in all patients. Fertility, when desired, is achieved in most cases but cryptorchidism not corrected early in life has a poor prognosis.

Keywords: Kallman's sundrome, anosmia, hypogonadism, amenorrhea

INTRODUCTION

In 1856, the link between anosmia and hypogonadism was established by Aureliano Maestre de San Juan, a Spanish physician [1, 2]. However, it was Franz Josef Kallmann, a German-American geneticist and his colleagues who in 1944 described the entity called Kallmann syndrome (KS) in full in a scientific paper publication [2, 3]. They described the familial nature of a syndrome comprising hypogonadotrophic hypogonadism and anosmia. The features result from defective migration of gonadotrophin-releasing hormone neurones from the medial olfactory placode epithelium into the anterior hypothalamus and failure of olfactory bulb genesis [3]. KS is usually inherited in an X-linked recessive manner but autosomal dominant and autosomal recessive forms do exist too. Patients with KS often present with delayed puberty, micropenis and cryptorchidism [4, 5].

KS belongs to group of conditions referred to as Hypogonadotropic hypogonadism (HH), with the only differentiating feature being the total or partial absence of sense of smell. This occurs in approximately 50% of HH cases [2, 5, 6].

Over twenty different genes have been implicated in causing KS through the disruption in the production of GnRH. The genes cover all forms of inheritance and no one gene defect has been shown to be common to all cases which makes genetic testing and prediction of inheritance pattern very challenging [2, 6].

EPIDEMIOLOGY

The prevalence of KS is still unknown. It is estimated at 1 out of 10,000 males with a lower rate in females. It is believed to be five times more common in males than females but there is no obvious genetic reason for this, even though two of the associated gene defects occur on the X-chromosome. The reported male predominance may not necessarily be a true gender imbalance but a reflection of the difficulty in diagnosing KS correctly especially in females with mild hypogonadism [2, 5, 6]. In addition primary amenorrhea in females may remain unexplored.

PATHOGENESIS

KS is a developmental disease that affects both the hormonal reproductive axis and the sense of smell. There is a developmental link between the reproductive and olfactory disorders: neuroendocrine cells producing the gonadotropin-releasing hormone that is deficient in the patients normally migrate from the nose to the forebrain along olfactory nerve fibers during embryonic life, and they most probably fail to do so in the patients. It is a hereditary disease with complex genetic transmission. KS can be caused by mutations in either of two different genes, *KAL1* and *FGFR1,* which have been found in approximately 20% of the affected individuals. Mutations in PROKR2 and PROK2, encoding prokineticin receptor-2 and prokineticin-2, have also been found in heterozygous, homozygous, and compound heterozygous states. These two genes are likely to be involved both in monogenic recessive and digenic/oligogenic KS transmission modes. Notably, mutations in any of the above-mentioned KS genes have been found in less than 30% of the KS patients, which indicates that other genes involved in the disease remain to be discovered [7, 8].

The most common modes of inheritance of KS are:

Autosomal dominant inheritance: Here dominant genetic disorders occur when only a single copy of an abnormal gene is necessary and sufficient to cause a particular disease. Therefore the risk of transmitting a dominant gene is the same for males and females and can be inherited from either of the parents. So the risk of transmitting the abnormal gene from an affected parent to the offspring is 50% for each pregnancy.

Autosomal recessive inheritance: The recessive genetic disorders also affect both sexes equally but differ from dominant inheritance in that a disease only occurs when an individual inherits two copies of an abnormal gene for the same trait, one from each parent. If an individual receives a normal gene and an abnormal gene for the disease, the person will be the disease carrier but will not show symptoms of that disease. Consanguineous marriages predispose to a higher risk of having children with a recessive genetic disorder than unrelated parents. The risk for two carrier parents to both pass the defective gene and have an affected child is 25% with each pregnancy. The risk to have a child who is a carrier like the parents is 50% with each pregnancy. The chance for a child to receive normal genes from both parents and be genetically normal for that particular trait is 25%.

X-linked inheritance: In this inheritance, the females with a mutation in a gene on the X-chromosome usually do not display symptoms of the disease linked to the genetic mutation since they have two X-chromosomes. The normal gene on the second X-chromosome compensates for the mutated one. However, since the males have only one X-chromosome that is inherited from their mother (hemizygosity), if they inherit an X-chromosome that contains a defective gene, they will develop the disease. Female carriers of an X-linked disorder have a 25% chance with each pregnancy to have a carrier daughter like themselves, a 25% chance to have a non-carrier daughter, a 25% chance to have a son affected with the disease and a 25% chance to have an unaffected son. If a male with an X-linked disorder is able to reproduce, he will pass the defective gene to all of his daughters who will then be carriers. A male cannot pass an X-linked gene to his sons.

Oligogenic inheritance: This is a newly recognized inheritance pattern in which mutations in more than one gene synergistically interact and function in an additive manner to cause a phenotypic disease. Both genes may have mutations in only one copy. Occasionally, one gene may have two mutations, each in a different allele they carry and the other may harbor a single mutation giving triallelic-digenic inheritance. About 10-15% of isolated GnRH deficiency patients have been shown to display this form of inheritance.

CLINICAL PRESENTATION

Kallmann syndrome typically combines severe hypogonadotropic hypogonadism with a complete absence of the sense of smell (anosmia). However, the degree of the hypogonadism and anosmia can vary greatly [2]. Variety of non-reproductive non-olfactory anomalies is in some significant proportion of KS patients (Table 1). These disorders include abnormal eye movements, congenital ptosis, abnormal visual spatial attention, hearing impairment agenesis of the corpus callosum, unilateral or bilateral, renal agenesis, cleft lip or palate, agenesis of one or several teeth, involuntary upper limb mirror movements and obesity.

Table 1. Clinical Features of Kallmann Syndrome

Reproductive features	Non-reproductive features
Amenorrhea	Anosmia Deafness Synkinesis Renal agenesis Dental anomalies Syndactyly Cleft lip or cleft palate Coloboma

Differential Diagnosis

Classic KS and idiopathic hypogonadotropic hypogonadism are rare genetic conditions that encompass the spectrum of isolated hypogonadotropic hypogonadism. Common feature in both conditions is presence of gonadotropin-releasing hormone (GnRH) deficiency. This is evidenced by their response to pulsatile GnRH therapy. Hypothalamic-pituitary function is normal in most patients, and hypothalamic-pituitary imaging shows no space-occupying lesions. KS is differentiated from spectrum by presence of either anosmia or severe hyposmia which in contrast to patients with idiopathic hypogonadotropic hypogonadism, whose sense of smell is normal.

Hypothalamo-hypophyseal dysfunction is the cause of growth retardation, genital hypoplasia and delayed puberty in CHARGE syndrome and may be confused with KS. By contrast, olfactory dysfunction is not present in CHARGE syndrome.

Other differential diagnosis of KS includes, constitutionally delayed puberty, neoplastic and inflammatory diseases. MRI imaging can exclude hypothalamic and pituitary tumors such as craniopharyngiomas or adenomas.

Management

Diagnosis

The diagnosis of KS is often made with substantial delay, despite clues in childhood such as anosmia, cryptorchidism and failure to enter puberty at the right time. Bone maturation and formation of longitudinal growth may occur at an age beyond 20 years. Concomitant deficits of other pituitary hormones should be excluded by history, clinical examination and laboratory findings.

There are two types of smell tests. One uses small bottles that have different substances in them; the other test uses "scratch and sniff" cards. Both tests use substances that have strong smells that most everyone knows, such as coffee. If the person being tested has a normal sense of smell, then another disorder besides Kallmann syndrome is present.

A physical examination will show whether undescended testes or small genitals are present in a male. A family history of KS would be an important clue to diagnosis. A blood test is done to measure the levels of luteinizing hormone (LH) and follicle stimulating hormone (FSH), as well as testosterone or estrogen. All these hormones are important for normal sexual development. Very low levels of these hormones mean there is a problem with either the hypothalalmus or the pituitary gland in the brain.

In KS, the lack of a sense of smell is due to the absence of structures called olfactory bulbs in the brain. A magnetic resonance imaging (MRI) scan of the head can show whether these structures are present or not.

The essential investigations in the diagnosis and confirmation of person with KS are listed with explanation in Table 2.

Table 2. Essential investigation in suspected case of Kallmann's Syndrome

Test	Explanation
1. Serum electrolytes	Normal serum electrolyte levels
2. Serum ferritin	Normal Serum ferritin levels. Measured to exclude haemochromatosis, an important cause of acquired hypogonadotropic hypogonadism.
3. Beta-human chorionic gonadotropin level	A must in patients with secondary amenorrhea to rule out pregnancy.
4. Serum (total or free) testosterone	Reduced serum level Measured to exclude hyperandrogenic disorders
5. Serum estradiol	Reduced serum level
6. Serum LH and FSH	Low- normal or reduced serum levels are low-normal. Measure to differentiate Kallmann 's syndrome primary gonadal dysfunction
7. Serum TSH and free thyroxine index	Normal serum levels Measured to exclude idiopathic hypogonadotropic hypogonadism with normal or low TSH level and a low serum free thyroxine level.
8. Serum insulin-like growth factor I and serum insulin-like growth factor binding protein 3	Normal serum levels Measured to exclude growth hormone deficiency in childhood
9. Early morning serum cortisol and plasma adrenocorticotropic hormone	Normal serum levels Measured to screen for adrenocortical insufficiency in patients with suspected idiopathic hypogonadotropic hypogonadism.
10. Serum prolactin	Normal serum levels Measured to exclude hyperprolactinemic conditions

Table 2. (Continued)

Test	Explanation
11. Brain MRI	Abnormal olfactory systems which consists of complete agenesis of olfactory bulbs and sulci, shallow olfactory sulci, or medial orientation of the olfactory sulci.
12. Transthoracic echocardiogram	Screening for congenital heart disease, which is present in a small proportion of Kallmann's syndrome patients.
13. Abdomino-pelvic ultrasound scan	Exclude unilateral renal agenesis, which affects a small proportion of patients
14. Bone densitometry by dual-energy radiographic absorptiometry (DXA)	Recommended for all hypogonadal patients to detect the presence of osteopenia or osteoporosis and to monitor the response of the skeleton to hormone replacement therapy.
15. Progestin-induced withdrawal bleeding:	KS patients are unlikely to have withdrawal bleeding because they do not have estrogen-primed endometrium.

Treatment

The treatment of KS aims first to initiate breast development, and secondly to achieve fertility. Hormone replacement therapy, usually with combined oestrogen and progesterone, is the treatment to stimulate the development of secondary sexual characteristics. For those desiring fertility, either gonadotropins or pulsatile GnRH can be used to achieve ovulation. The treatments restore fertility in a vast majority of affected individuals [2].

Psychotherapy: Behavioral modification and psychological counseling may benefit individuals with KS.

Hormone replacement therapy: Hormone replacement theray is given to all postpubertal-age patients with KS in the absence of contraindications.

Other medical therapies: Should be individualised to treat associated conditions like osteoporosis, adrenocortical insufficiency, congenital heart disease, and neurologic disorders. Additional therapies to restore fertility are based on patient need e.g., Clomiphene citrate.

Surgical treatment: Assisted reproductive technologies should be used on KS patients, who in spite of the use of hormone replacement therapy, have infertility problem. Those with congenital heart disease, cleft lips and palate will benefit from corrective surgery.

Pre-Conceptional Counselling

When autosomal dominant transmission is suspected, the patient and partner should receive genetic counselling before fertility-inducing treatment. This comprises an explanation of the 50% theoretical risk of transmitting the disease. In autosomal recessive forms, in absence of consanguinity, the risk of the disease transmission to offspring is very low. Male patients with X-linked Kallmann's syndrome should be counselled of the automatic transmission of the mutation to their daughters. Therefore genetic counselling of their daughters from the puberty age is very necessary. When KS patients have oligogenic inheritance, genetic counselling is difficult because the transmission risk is variable.

PROGNOSIS

KS patients can survive for prolonged period when there is no co-existing life-threatening conditions. Fertility can be restored in most of the patients. Though, KS was initially thought to be a permanent disorder, there were reported cases of KS patients who experienced spontaneous complete recovery of gonadal function [8]. Some other cases experienced complete recovery of gonadal function when the precipitating factors are corrected. However some patients with congenital heart disease or neurologic manifestations may experience a shortened lifespan. Unless it is detected early and adequately treated, adrenocortical insufficiency is usually fatal. Osteoporosis increases the risk of fracture, which may jeopardize patient's survival and quality of life.

PREVENTION OF KALLMANN SYNDROME

Though majority of KS cases are sporadic, the familial form of the disease can be prevented through avoidance of consanguineous marriages, genetic counselling and testing of individuals with the disease trait. Family planning and preconceptional counselling of the couple with KS trait is necessary to help limit their number of children and prepare the couple on the possible outcomes of each pregnancy. Prenatal diagnosis of the fetuses with KS will further help the couple decide on whether to terminate the pregnancy, especially if there are associated major congenital fetal anomalies, when they are in countries with liberal abortion laws. For the couple who decide to keep the pregnancy, prenatal diagnosis will help them prepare for the delivery and follow up of the child.

CONCLUSION

The KS combines hypogonadotropic hypogonadism (HH) with anosmia. This is a clinically and genetically heterogeneous disease. KAL1, encoding the extracellular glycoprotein anosmin-1, is responsible for the X-chromosome-linked recessive form of the disease. Four forms of Kallmann syndrome, designated types 1 through 4, have been identified by researchers. The four types are each characterized by hypogonadotropic hypogonadism and an impaired sense of smell. Additional features, such as a cleft palate, seem to occur only in types 1 and 2. Treatment of KS is in that of the hypogonadism. There is currently no treatment for olfactory deficit. Hormone replacement therapies are used to stimulate the development of secondary sexual characteristics at the time of puberty, and later to induce fertility.

References

[1] Maestre de San Juan, Aureliano. Teratolagia: falta total de los nervios olfactorios con anosmia en un individuo en quien existia una atrofia congenita de los testiculos y miembro viril. *El Siglo Médico* 1856; 3: 211–221.

[2] Dodé, Catherine, and Jean-Pierre Hardelin. “Kallmann syndrome.” *European Journal of Human Genetics* 2009; 17(2): 139-146.

[3] Kallmann F. J., Schönfeld W. A., Barrera S. E., The genetic aspects of primary eunuchoidism. *American Journal of Mental Deficiency* 1944; 48: 203–236.

[4] Valdes-Socin, H., Reproduction, smell, and neurodevelopmental disorders: genetic defects in different hypogonadotropic hypogonadal syndromes. *Frontiers in Endocrinology* 2014; 5: 109.

[5] Schwanzel-Fukuda, M., Bick, D., Pfaff, D. W., (1989). Luteinizing hormone-releasing hormone (LHRH)-expressing cells do not migrate normally in an inherited hypogonadal (Kallmann) syndrome. *Brain Res Mol Brain Res.* 1989; 6 (4): 311-26.

[6] Deeb, A., Robertson, A., MacColl, G., Bouloux, P. M., Gibson, M., Winyard, P. J., ... and Cheetham, T. D., (2001). Multicystic dysplastic kidney and Kallmann's syndrome: a new association?. *Nephrology Dialysis Transplantation* 2001; *16*(6), 1170-1175.

[7] Dodé, Catherine, Luis Teixeira, Jacqueline Levilliers, Corinne Fouveaut, Philippe Bouchard, Marie-Laure Kottler, James Lespinasse et al. “Kallmann syndrome: mutations in the genes encoding prokineticin-2 and prokineticin receptor-2.” *PLoS Genet* 2, no. 10 (2006): e175.

[8] Dode C., Hardelin J. P., Kallmann syndrome, *Eur. Journal of Human Gentics* 2009;17: 139–146.

SECTION III: SECONDARY AMENORRHEA

In: Amenorrhea
Editor: Oliver Chukwujekwu Ezechi

ISBN: 978-1-63484-778-0

Chapter 11

ASHERMAN'S SYNDROME

Tinuade Abimbola Oyebode
Department of Obstetrics and Gynaecology, University of Jos, Jos, Nigeria

ABSTRACT

Asherman's syndrome is a condition characterized by endometrial adhesions usually following dilation and curettage. Trauma to the basal layer of the endometrium causes intrauterine adhesions which obliterate the cavity in varying degrees and presents with secondary amenorrhea. These abound in unsafe abortions, pelvic infections and retained products of conception. Caesarean section, myomectomy, foreign bodies, irradiation, schistosomiasis and genital tuberculosis cause severe adhesions which are difficult to treat. About 40% of patients undergoing repeated dilatation and curettage developed Asherman's syndrome, but a single curettage often underlies the condition. Hysteroscopy is the gold standard for diagnosis. Various classification systems were developed considering amount of functioning residual endometrium, menstrual pattern, obstetric history and uterine adhesions location and severity. Fertility and menstruation may be restored using operative hysteroscopy for adhesiolysis. Foleys catheters, IUCD, hyaluronic acid gel barrier, antibiotic prophylaxis, sequential estrogen/progestin to stimulate endometrial growth and prevent recurrence are options. Mild adhesions can be successfully treated, while extensive endometrial obliteration and tubal ostia occlusion may require several surgeries or be uncorrectable. Patients conceiving after treatment of intrauterine adhesion are at increased risk for abnormal placentation, premature delivery, abortions and uterine rupture. To prevent occurrence of Asherman's syndrome, Misoprostol use is safer for managing incomplete/missed abortions, retained placenta and postpartum hemorrhage, followed by manual vacuum aspiration.

Keywords: Asherman's syndrome, amenorrhea, abortion, endometritis

INTRODUCTION

Asherman's syndrome is an acquired gynaecological condition which is characterized by endometrial and/or cervical adhesions or fibrosis. The condition typically follows vigorous dilation and curettage (D&C) procedures but can also inflict any woman undergoing any form of intrauterine procedure. It is also known as intrauterine adhesions (IUA), amenorrhea traumatica, endometrial sclerosis, intrauterine scarring, Fritsch syndrome and intrauterine synechiae [1]. The condition was first described in 1894 by Heinrich Fritsch [2], but was further characterized by the Israeli gynecologist Joseph Asherman's in 1948 [2, 3]. In its severe forms, the condition is responsible for extensive morbidity including permanent infertility, unlike the mild forms which are thought to be under diagnosed because symptoms are mild.

EPIDEMIOLOGY

The true incidence of uterine synechiae is not known, however it is estimated that 25% of dilatation and curettage performed between the first and fourth weeks post-partum are said to develop intrauterine synechiae [4, 5], while 30.9% of those performed for missed miscarriages [6], and 6.4% performed for incomplete miscarriages also develop the condition [7]. It is also estimated that about 40% of patients undergoing repeated curettage developed Asherman's syndrome. In missed miscarriages, the time between fetal demise and curettage may increase adhesion formation due to fibroblastic activity. The risk increases with number of procedures (16% after one D&C and 32% after 3 or more D&Cs) [8]. However, a single curettage often underlies the condition in many cases. Studies have found synechiae in 1.5% of women undergoing hysterosalpingography, and 5- 39% women with recurrent miscarriage [9].

Pathogenesis

The endometrium lines the uterine cavity and is composed of the functional layer which is shed off during menstruation and a basal layer beneath it that helps regenerate the functional layer of the endometrium. Trauma to the endometrium basal layer, typically after dilatation and curettage procedures, causes development of intrauterine scars/adhesions that obliterate the cavity in varying degrees by causing the anterior and posterior walls of the uterus to adhere to each other. The scar tissues are usually avascular and even in the presence of very few scars; the endometrium may fail to respond to endogenous oestrogen causing patients to present with secondary amenorrhea. Asherman's syndrome abound in environment of unsafe abortions, severe pelvic infections, puerperal sepsis, retained products of conception and other conditions that warrant uterine evacuation. Caesarean section, myomectomy, packing of the uterus to arrest post-partum haemorrhage and foreign body such as an Intrauterine Contraceptive Device, irradiation, schistosomiasis and endometritis from genital tuberculosis cause severe intrauterine adhesions that is difficult to treat. It has been reported that 88% of AS cases occur after a D&C is performed on a recently pregnant uterus, following a missed or incomplete miscarriage, birth, or during an elective termination (abortion) to remove retained products of conception. This is therefore a condition that is found more in places where reproductive health services are still inadequate [10].

Data regarding pathophysiology are still limited but evaluation of endometrial glandular cells revealed significant sub-cellular modifications including ribosome loss, mitochondria swelling, vascular closure and hypoxic cellular modifications [11]. An impaired vascularity of both endometrium and myometrium has been demonstrated by using pelvic angiography in patients with dense intrauterine adhesions [12]. Some workers also demonstrated high impedance of spiral artery and propose that this could explain the reduced endometrial receptivity and regeneration observed in Asherman's [13]. It has also been suggested that adhesion related cytokines such as b-fibroblast growth factor, platelet derived growth factor and transforming growth factor type 1 may be involved in the pathogenesis of intrauterine synechiae [14].

Although not clearly identified, a possible genetic factor could explain why certain patients show more frequent adhesions incidence and recurrence, or why IUA adhesions can develop even without any surgical trauma or trigger event [15].

There are three types of pathology in Asherman's syndrome. The most common pathology is avascular fibrous strands joining the uterine walls. Occasionally, this condition may be accompanied by deep adenomyosis and myometrium may be present in the bands of adhesion. In this type, the muscular adhesions are denser and indicate a deficient endometrial basalis and a poorer prognosis. The other cases have only a sclerotic, atrophic endometrium and thus they carry the worst prognosis [16].

Classification Systems

The evaluation of the extent of the adhesions, determines the most appropriate therapeutic regimen, and predicts the result of treatment of Asherman's syndrome requires a proper classification. An ideal classification system should include a comprehensive description of the adhesions, grade it in terms of severity and in addition provide a practical guide to the achievement of optimum treatment and likely outcome. Various classification systems have been proposed, with each attempting to find the most accurate classification for Asherman's syndrome. Various classification systems were developed to describe Asherman's syndrome, some taking into account the amount of functioning residual endometrium, menstrual pattern, obstetric history and other factors which are thought to play a role in determining the prognoses. With the advent of techniques which allow visualization of the uterus, classification systems were developed to take into account the location and severity of adhesions inside the uterus. This is useful as mild cases with adhesions restricted to the cervix may present with amenorrhea and infertility, showing that symptoms alone do not necessarily reflect severity. Other patients may have no adhesions but amenorrhea and infertility due to a sclerotic atrophic endometrium. The latter form has the worst prognosis [17].

The ideal classification system should include a comprehensive description of the adhesions which should be graded in terms of severity and ought to provide a practical guide for clinicians to achieve optimum treatment and likely outcome. Since Asherman's original description, there have been many attempts to find the most accurate classification for IUAs.

Table 1. Hysterosalpingographic classification of Toeff and Ballas

Classification	Condition
Type 1	Atresia of the internal ostium, without concomitant corporal adhesions
Type 2	Stenosis of internal ostium, causing almost complete occlusion without concomitant corporal adhesions
Type 3	Multiple small adhesions in the internal ostium isthmic region
Type 4	Supra isthmic diaphragm causing complete separation of the main cavity form its lower segment
Type 5	Atresia of the internal ostium with concomitant corporeal adhesions.

Table 2. Classification of Asherman's syndrome by March et al. 1978

Classification	Condition
Mild	Filmy adhesion occupying less than one-quarter of uterine cavity. Ostial areas and upper fundus minimally involved or clear.
Moderate	One-fourth to three fourth of cavity involved. Ostial areas and upper fundus partially involved. No agglutination of uterine walls
Severe	More than three fourth of cavity involved. Occlusion of both ostial area and upper fundus. Agglutination of uterine walls

Toeff and Ballas Classification

Toeff and Ballas in 1978 were the first to classify Asherman's syndrome (Table 1). Hysterosalpingography findings was the basis of their classification [18].

This classification is still used for its simplicity although it is considered insufficiently prognostic [19].

March, Israel and March 1978 classification

March and colleague, late in 1978 introduced for the first time a hysteroscopic classification of Asherman's Syndrome (Table 2) [20]. This classification is still been used because of its simplicity, although it is insufficiently prognostic.

Valle and Sciarra's 1988 Classification [21]

This classification system utilised both hysterecopy assessment and HSG findings. Adhesions were classified as mild, moderate, or severe according to hysteroscopic assessment and extent of occlusion as partial or total at hysterosalpingram (Table 3).

American Society for Reproductive Medicine Classification 1988

The American Society for Reproductive Medicine (ASRM) is a modification of March 1978 classification system (table 4). In addition to considering the extent of cavity involvement and types of adhesion, as in the March system, it included menstrual pattern of the patients, potentially offering some prognostic information [22]. It is an objective scoring system for classification of intrauterine adhesions as it correlated the menstrual history with hysteroscopic and hysterosalpingography findings. The grade and description of the ASRM classification system are shown in Table 2 below.

The European Society for Hysteroscopy Classification

The European Society of Hysteroscopy (ESH) adopted the classification developed at the Hysteroscopy Training Centre in the Netherlands by Wamsteker [23]. The classification distinguishes the severity of Asherman's syndrome based on the thickness of adhesion band, patency of the tubal ostia and extent of uterine cavity obliteration (Table 5).

Table 3. Valle and Sciarra 1988 classification

Degree	Description
Mild	Filmy adhesions composed of basal endometrium producing partial or complete uterine cavity occlusion
Moderate	Fibromuscular adhesions that are characteristically thick, still covered by endometrium that may bleed on division, partially or totally occluding the uterine cavity
Severe	Composed of connective tissue with no endometrial lining and likely to bleed upon division, partially or totally occluding the uterine cavity.

Table 4. The American Society for Reproductive Medicine classification of intrauterine adhesions, 1988

Extent of cavity involved	<1/3	1/3 – 2/3	>2/3
	1	2	4
Type of adhesions	Filmy	Filmy and Dense	Dense
	1	2	4
Menstrual pattern	Normal	Hypomenorrhoea	Amenorrhea
	0	2	4
Prognostic classification		HSG[a] Score	Hysteroscopy Score
Stage l		(Mild)	1-4
Stage ll		(Moderate)	5-8
Stage lll		(Severe)	9-12

Donnez and Nisolle 1994 Classification [24]

The classification primarily use the location of the adhesions and rate of pregnancy post treatment as the basis. In this system Asherman's syndrome is classified into 6 grades (Table 6). Hysteroscopy or HSG are used for assessment.

Clinical Presentation

The presentation of AS varies, most times the patients present with the complications of the condition. Asherman's Syndrome is known to affect women of all races and ages equally, suggesting that there is no underlying genetic predisposition for its development [25]. Depending on the degree of severity, AS may result in infertility, secondary amenorrhea, recurrent spontaneous abortions, cryptomenorrhoea with cyclical pain from trapped blood, and future obstetric complications [26]. If left untreated, the obstruction of menstrual flow resulting from adhesions can lead to bleeding into the peritoneal cavity leading to endometriosis with its attendant complications in some cases [27].

Investigation

Clinical Evaluation

There must be a high index of suspicion and the history of events proceeding complaints must be sought. History of preceding pregnancy must be sought as well as outcomes, duration, interventions and complications. In order To rule out other conditions the history should seek information about if patient have attained secondary sexual characteristics, has a normal height and had previously attained menarche and had previously experienced normal monthly menstruation. The history is usually typical of a pregnancy event, commonly an abortion or postpartum haemorrhage, followed by uterine evacuation with or without severe sepsis followed by secondary amenorrhea. The other gynaecological and obstetric conditions like myomectomy and caesarean section that could predispose to Asherman's syndrome may also be elicited from the history. Some patients may have cyclical bleeds but quantity of effluent is minimal and the numbers of days are also much less than previously, while some women with intrauterine synechiae in mild forms have normal monthly periods. Others who have cervical synechiae with some intact endometrium may experience some degree of cyclical abdominal pain on account of cryptomenorrhoea.

Recurrent abortions and infertility can also be the presenting symptoms, but history to rule out other causes of secondary amenorrhea must be obtained.

Physical examination may not yield much, but should be done exhaustively to exclude other causes of secondary amenorrhea in uncertain cases. It should basically include height and weight, Body Mass Index, hair distribution, Tanner staging, seeking anterior neck masses and cardiovascular examination. Abdominal examination may yield an enlarged uterus if there is hematometra, while cervical examination may reveal cervical stenosis and other forms of acquired gynaetresia that may have followed the preceding procedure.

Table 5. European Society of Hysteroscopy classification system

Grade	Description
I	Thin or filmy adhesions easily ruptured by hysteroscope sheath alone, cornual areas normal
II	Singular firm adhesions connecting separate parts of the uterine cavity, visualization of both tubal ostia possible, cannot be ruptured by hysteroscope sheath alone;
	IIa - Occluding adhesions only in the region of the internal cervical OS. Upper uterine cavity normal;
III	Multiple firm adhesions connecting separate parts of the uterine cavity, unilateral obliteration of ostial areas of the tubes;
	IIIa - Extensive scarring of the uterine cavity wall with amenorrhea or hypomenorrhea;
	IIIb - Combination of III and IIIa;
IV	Extensive firm adhesions with agglutination of the uterine walls. Both tubal ostial areas occluded

Table 6. Donnes and Nisolle classification system

Grade	Description
1	Central adhesions
	a. Thin filmy adhesions (endometrial adhesions)
	b. Myofibrous (connective adhesions)
II	Marginal adhesions (always myofibrous or connective)
	a. Wedge like projection
	b. Obliteration of one horn
III	Uterine cavity absent on HSG
	a. Occlusion of the internal os (upper cavity normal)
	b. Extensive agglutination of uterine walls (absence of uterine cavity - true Asherman's)

Laboratory and Clinical Investigation

Blood tests may not yield much but may be carried out to detect tuberculosis or schistosomiasis in areas where the prevalence may be high. Ultrasound is unreliable for diagnosis but may reveal an enlarged uterus with features suggesting a collection. Hormonal assays are same as in normal people except where there are coexisting morbidities. Weekly serum progesterone assays and values >3ng/ml that are not associated with menstrual bleeds are indicative of Asherman's syndrome. Carrying out progesterone challenge test or combined oestrogen progesterone challenge tests will not induce bleeds in this patient considering that the ovarian function is not affected in this condition. Sonohysterography or hysterosalpingography can be carried out, especially in low resource environments that still lack hysteroscopy but have X-ray and Ultrasound machines. These will reveal extent of scarification by outlining the parts of the uterus and cervix that have filling defects [28].

Differential Diagnosis

Although the history of pregnancy and evacuation of the uterus is classical in these women, other causes of secondary amenorrhea should be ruled out. These could as well coexist with Asherman's syndrome. These include the use of drugs like progestogen containing drugs and contraception, hormonal abnormalities like Prolactinaemia, thyroid and adrenal dysfunction, polycystic ovarian disorders which can be ruled out with the corresponding hormonal assays. The amenorrhea associated with waning ovarian function of the climacteric should also be considered and can be ruled out with history and hormonal assays which can reveal elevated FSH levels and reduced estradiol levels. Anorexia nervosa, severe anxiety and chronic debilitating illnesses can also cause secondary amenorrhea. Taking a good clinical history and physical examination and conducting needful evaluations like HIV screening among others will distinguish these from secondary amenorrhea from Asherman's syndrome.

Treatment

In the past, different approaches have been used to treatment Asherman's syndrome, but successful treatment methods relied on the breakdown of the adhesions, prevention of the recurrence of adhesion and restoration of some degree of normal-appearing and functioning endometrium. The treatment of Asherman's syndrome is summarized in Table 7 below.

Adhesiolysis

Fertility may sometimes be restored by adhesiolysis (removal of intrauterine adhesions), but severity of the initial trauma and other individual patient factors are prognostic factors. Adhesiolysis can be carried out in various ways and some of the methods are now historic in parts of the world that have better capacity than the low resource settings.

Table 7. Treatment strategy and methods for Asherman's syndrome

Treatment strategy	Mode of treatment
Adhesiolysis	Dilatation and curettage Hysteroscopy Hysterotomy
Recurrence prevention	Intrauterine device Uterine balloon stent Foley's catheter Anti-adhesion barriers
Restoring normal endometrium	Hormonal treatment Stem cells
Post-operative assessment	Clinical evaluation Diagnostic hysteroscopy Ultrasound with contrast

Hysterotomy

Before the advent of operative hysteroscopy some cases of Asherman's syndrome treatment using an open-surgery approach with transfundal separation of scarring uterine walls have been described, with varying success. However in some cases an adequate restoration of menstruation and fertility was obtained [29]. Hysterotomy procedure for adhesiolysis has been superseded by hysteroscopic techniques, It is important to known that it may still have a place in very complex situation, when the hysteroscopic approach is not possible or unlikely to succeed. The risk associated with the procedure and possibility of failure to achieve desired result of cavity restoration, menstruation and or fertility may not be obtained. However in desperate attempts to address patients complains, blind adhesiolysis procedures are sometimes carried out in some centers where hysteroscopy is not available, with the attendant risks of possible uterine perforation. It is however largely an obsolete procedure in the treatment of Asherman's syndrome.

Dilatation and Curettage

This is carried suboptimal but has a place especially in low income settings where hysteroscopy is not available. It is also a blind procedure and complications like uterine perforation and cervical incompetence can occur following it. There can also be residual adhesions and persistence of symptoms.

Hysteroscopy

Adhesiolysis with the use of the Operative hysteroscopy is used for visual inspection of the uterine cavity during evaluation for Asherman's and as well for adhesion dissection at the same sitting. This is the gold standard for evaluation and treatment of Asherman's syndrome by adhesiolysis. Fertility and menstruation may be restored using operative hysteroscopy for visual inspection and adhesiolysis. It must be performed by an experienced surgeon and the procedure must be carefully performed in order to avoid new scars and further exacerbation of the condition. However, hysteroscopy is yet to become a routine gynaecological procedure and only very few centers in resource constrained settings have the required equipment and skilled manpower. Adhesion dissection can be technically difficult and must be performed with care in order to not create new scars and further exacerbate the condition. In more severe cases, adjunctive measures such as laparoscopy are used in conjunction with hysteroscopy as a protective measure against uterine perforation. Micro scissors are usually used to cut adhesions while electro cauterization is not recommended as it tends to predispose to reoccurrence of scar formation [30]. Complications of hysteroscopic surgery are uncommon. When they occur, they may include bleeding, perforation of the uterus, and pelvic infection.

Prevention of Adhesion Recurrence

Recurrences of adhesions post adhesiolysis are common. The rate of reformation of intrauterine adhesions after adhesiolysis remains high with rates ranging from 3.1% to 23.5% reported in the literature [31, 32]. However these adhesions tend to be thin and filmy usually [33]. To forestall the recurrence of the adhesions various techniques has been adopted to prevent the walls of the uterus re-apposing before the endometrium is restored.

Intrauterine Device (IUD)

The use of IUD to prevent adhesion recurrence was one of the first attempts to be documented in literature [34]. This was based on the premise that an IUD could help physiological endometrial regeneration by separating the anterior and posterior uterine walls. Several authors reported good results [35], but there are conflicts in available data with uncertainty about type and size of IUD to be utilized. Vesce et al. used a copper IUD with good results in 48 women with functional amenorrhea. In a short follow-up after the insertion of the IUD, a significant number of women regained a regular menses [36]. Other authors allude that Copper IUD induced inflammatory factors worsen endometrial injury [37]. Touguc et al. found no difference in adhesion reformation among women randomized to receive IUD device, estrogens treatment or no treatment after hysteroscopic septum resection [38]. The Levonorgestrel-releasing IUD should not be used for his suppressing effect on the endometrium [39]. The T-shaped IUD seems to be too tiny to guarantee a stable separation between the uterine walls, while the Lippes loop in account of it is peculiar trapezoidal shape, was considered the most adequate device to prevent adhesion albeit it is no longer available in the global market.

Intrauterine Balloon Stent

This is silicon made, triangular intrauterine stent which fits the normal triangular shape of the uterine cavity has been described for use as a mechanical method to prevent adhesions recurrence (Cook medical Inc, Bloomington, USA) Good fertility outcomes were achieved among 1240 patients treated using intrauterine stent with pregnancy rate of 61.6% and spontaneous miscarriage rate of 15.6% [40]. No data about IUA recurrence was reported. The author recommends prophylactic broad-spectrum antibiotic until the stent remains inside uterine cavity. In a recent cohort retrospective study of 107 patients with Asherman's syndrome, the use of intrauterine balloon stent, compared with IUD and hyaluronic acid, resulted in significantly higher reduction of adhesions recurrence rate [41] but data about its safety and efficacy seem still insufficient.

Foley Catheter

The Foley catheter was one of first mechanical devices used to separate the uterine walls preventing the recurrence of the intrauterine adhesions. It can be left for 7 -14 days as an adjuct to adhesiolysis. Some researchers tried covering it with fresh amnion graft and had good outcomes [42]. The use of Foley's catheter which was left for ten days in situ was found by some to have better conception rates when compared with women who had IUD which was left for three cycles (33.9% versus 22.5%), while 81% had restoration of their normal menstrual pattern [43]. There are however no randomized controlled trials demonstrating superiority of the Foley's catheter efficacy in the prevention of recurrent adhesions. The Foleys catheter is associated with discomfort, ascending infection and uterine perforation while the advantage is that it is left for a shorter time in situ.

Hyaluronic Acid and Other Anti-Adhesion Barriers

Hyaluronic acid is a widespread component of human tissues involved in biological functions such as mechanical support, cell migration and proliferation. Hyaluronic acid derivatives have been adopted in gynaecological surgery to prevent intraperitoneal and intrauterine adhesions [44, 45]. It generates a temporary barrier between organs which mechanically prevents adhesions formation and they influence peritoneal tissue repair by increasing proliferation rates of mesothelial cells [46]. More recently, the autocross-linked hyaluronic acid (Hyalobarrier©) is now available. It is a highly viscous gel formed by the autocross-linked condensation of hyaluronic acid which has in recent systematic review confirmed that it can prevent intraperitoneal adhesion after laparoscopic myomectomy and intrauterine adhesions after hysteroscopy procedure [47]. Others include Seprafilm© (sodium hyaluronate and carboxymethylcellulose), carboxymethylcellulose hyaluronic acid and alginate carboxymethylcellulose hyaluronic acid [48].

Restoration of Normal Endometrium

Restoration of normal endometrial tissue within the uterine cavity is the short term goals of the treatment of Asherman's syndrome, with restoration of menstruation and pregnancy as the ultimate goal. The restoration of normal uterine endometrium can be achieved either through medical therapy or stem cell transfer [49].

Medical Therapy

Several authors have proposed hormonal administration [50], although there is no consensus about timing of administration (preoperative and/or postoperative) and the type of regimen (oestradiol or combined oestradiol and progesterone). The general idea is to encourage fast growth of any residual endometrium immediately after surgery with the dual purpose of preventing new scar formation and restoring a normal uterine environment. March et al. suggested a treatment with micronized oestradiol, 2 mg twice daily for 30–60 days and medroxyprogesterone acetate 10 mg per day at last 5 days of oestrogen therapy [51]. Others prescribed estradiolvalerate 4 mg per day for 4 weeks and medroxyprogesterone acetate, 10 mg per day at last two week of treatment [52]. The intravaginal use of sildenafil citrate was documented as possible pharmacological treatment to restore endometrial thickness. Endometrial thickness improved and both women become pregnant after the first treatment cycle [53]. Most of the time these are used in conjunction with prophylactic antibiotics in the post-operative period.

Stem Cells and Endometrial Regeneration

Adult endometrial tissue contains epithelial progenitor cells and mesenchymal/stromal cells and endometrial tissue had an intrinsic capacity of regeneration which normally occurs after menstruation and delivery [54]. These cells can be used to regenerate endometrial tissue in cases of dysfunctional or atrophic endometrium and a Asherman's treated with autologous stem cells isolated from the women's own bone marrow was described [55].

Post-Operative Assessment

Presently, there is no clear consensus about follow up management but post-treatment assessment of the uterine cavity is recommended one-two months after the initial surgery [57]. Ultrasound, HSG and hysteroscopy are the most common follow-up methods. Ultrasound can measure endometrial thickness and assess normal endometrial development during menstrual cycle. HSG will check tubal patency in addition and can help resolve thin adhesions at the same sitting. Hysteroscopy is however the only method that allows an accurate estimation of adhesion recurrence. Timely recognition of any recurrence of adhesions is essential to provide the best prognosis, thus the most treatment protocols include a follow-up to assess endometrial restoration after the surgery.

Prognosis

Mild to moderate adhesions can be successfully treated while extensive endometrial obliteration, occlusion of tubal ostia and deep endometrial/myometrial trauma may require several surgeries or be uncorrectable. If the uterine cavity is adhesion free but ostia remain obliterated, IVF is an option.

For those who do not desire pregnancy, haematometra could re occur and this can lead to endometriosis with its attendant challenges. However, patients who successfully carry pregnancy after treatment have increased risk of abortions, abnormal placentation including placenta accreta, placenta increta, placenta percreta and placenta praevia. The risk of placenta praevia reduces when most of the adhesions are removed. Other problems include second-trimester pregnancy loss, cervical incompetence, premature delivery, abnormal foetal lie, intrauterine growth restriction, vasa praevia and uterine rupture. Women under 35 years have better outcomes.

Prevention

Considering that Asherman's Syndrome is known to be associated with curettage of the uterus either in early pregnancy or post-partum, this procedure can be restricted since there are medical options that are available with fewer complications. The drug Misoprostol is useful in evacuation of the uterus in cases of incomplete, induced and missed abortions and is equally effective in management of retained placenta and post-partum hemorrhage. These drugs should be considered in these conditions, since women did not develop intrauterine synechiae in cases of medical evacuation with misoprostol, while 7.7% of those undergoing curettage did. Immediate evacuation following fetal death and the use of hysteroscopic surgery instead of curettage could have better outcomes. Manual vacuum aspiration is a better option than curettage especially in resource constrained settings, even though some women have developed intrauterine synechiae following its use.

Conclusion

Asherman's syndrome remains a disorder with varying degrees and variants of morbidities. Obtaining optimal treatment outcomes are still challenging and emphasis should be placed on the prevention of this condition among women in the reproductive age group. This calls for training in essential obstetric care for health workers attending to women's health issues.

References

[1] Palter, S. "High Rates of Endometriosis in Patients with Intrauterine Synechiae (Asherman's Syndrome)." *Fertility and Sterility*, 86 (null), S471–S471. doi:10.1016/j.fertnstert.2005.07.1239.

[2] Fritsch, H. Ein Fall von volligem Schwaund der Gebormutterhohle nach Auskratzung. *Zentralbl Gynaekol*, 1894, 18, 1337-1342.

[3] Asherman, JG. Amenorrhea traumatica (atretica). *J Obstet Gynaecol Br Emp*, 1948, 55, 23-30 33.

[4] Shokeir, TA; Fawzy, M; Tatongy, M. The nature of intrauterine adhesions following reproductive hysteroscopic surgery as determined by early and late follow-up hysteroscopy: clinical implications. *Arch Gynecol Obstet*, 2008, 277, 423–427.

[5] Fedele, L; Bianchi, S; Frontino, G. Septums and synechiae: approaches to surgical correction. *Clin Obstet Gynecol*, 2006, 49, 767-788.

[6] Adoni, A; Palti, Z; Milwidsky, A; Dolberg, M. The incidence of intrauterine adhesions following spontaneous abortion. *Int J Fertil*, 1982, 27(2), 117-8.

[7] Schenker, JG; Margalioth, EJ. Intra-uterine adhesions: an updated appraisal. *Fertility Sterility*, 1982, 37, 593-610.

[8] Friedler, S; Margalioth, EJ; Karfka, I; Yaffe, H. Incidence of post-abortion intrauterine adhesions evaluated by hysteroscopy-a prospective study. *Hum Reprod*, 1993, 8, 442-4.

[9] Ventolini, G; Zhang, M; Gruber, J. Hysteroscopy in the evaluation of patients with recurrent pregnancy loss: a cohort study in a primary care population. *Surg Endosc*, 2004, 18, 1782-1784.

[10] Klein, SM; Garcia, C-R. "Asherman's syndrome: a critique and current review." *Fertility and Sterility*, 1973, 24 (9), 722–735.

[11] Chen, Y; Chang, Y; Yao, S. Role of angiogenesis in endometrial repair of patients with severe intrauterine adhesion. *Int J Clin Exp Pathol*, 2013, 15, 1343-1350.

[12] Polishuk, WZ; Kohane, S. Intrauterine adhesions: diagnosis and therapy. *Obstet Gynecol Digest,* 1966, 8, 41.

[13] Malhotra, N; Bahadur, A; Kalaivani, M; Mittal, S. Changes in endometrial receptivity in women with Asherman's syndrome undergoing hysteroscopic adhesiolysis.

[14] Tao, Z; Duan, H. Expression of adhesion-related cytokines in the uterine fluid after transcervical resection of adhesion.
[15] Yu, D; Wong, YM; Cheong, Y; Xia, E; Li, TC. Asherman syndrome-one century later. *Fertil Steril*, 2008, 89, 759-779.
[16] Foix, A; Bruno, RO; Davison, T; Lema, B. The pathology of post curettage adhesions. *Am. J. Obstet. Gynecol.*, 1966, 96, 1027-1033.
[17] Asherman's syndrome. From Wikipedia, the free encyclopedia.
[18] Available at: https://en.wikipedia.org/wiki/Asherman%27s_syndrome# Classification.
[19] Toaff, R; Ballas, S. Traumatic hypomenorrhea-amenorrhea (Asherman' syndrome). *Fertil Steril*, 1978, 30, 379–387.
[20] Nasr, AL; Al-Inany, HG; Thabet, SM; Aboulghar, MA. Clinicohysteroscopic scoring system of intrauterine adhesions. *Gynecol Obstet Invest*, 2000, 50, 178-181.
[21] March, CM; Israel, R; March, AD. Hysteroscopic management of intrauterine adhesions. *Am. J. Obstet. Gynecol.*, 1978, 130, 653-657.
[22] Valle, RF; Sciarra, JJ. intrauterine adhesions: Hysteroscopic diagnosis, classification, treatment, and reproductive outcome. *American Journal of Obstetrics and Gynecology*, 1988, 158, 1459-1470.
[23] The American Fertility Society. The American Fertility Society classification of adnexal adhesions, distal tubal occlusion, tubal occlusion secondary to tubal ligation, tubal pregnancies, Mullerian anomalies and intrauterine adhesions. *Fertil. Steril.*, 1988, 49, 944-955.
[24] Wamsteker, K; De Block, S. Diagnostic hysteroscopy: technique and documentation. In: Sutton C, Diamond M, eds. Endoscopic surgery for gynecologists. London: WB Saunders, 1998, 511–24.
[25] Donnez, J; Nisolle, M. Hysteroscopic Adhesiolysis of Intrauterine Adhesions (Asherman Syndrome). In: Donnez J, editor. London, England: Parthenon Publishing Group, 1994.
[26] Schenker, JG; Margalioth, EJ. "Intra-uterine adhesions: an updated appraisal." *Fertility and Sterility*, 1982, 37 (5), 593–610.
[27] Valle, RF; Sciarra, JJ. "Intrauterine adhesions: Hystreoscopic diagnosis, classification, treatment and reproductive outcome." *Am J Obstet*, 1988, 158 (6Pt1), 1459–1470.
[28] Palter, S. "High Rates of Endometriosis in Patients with Intrauterine Synechiae (Asherman's Syndrome)." *Fertility and Sterility*, 2005, 86 (null), S471–S471.
[29] Kenneth, F. Trofatter, Jr. Asherman's Syndrome: Diagnosis, Treatment, and Prevention. Available at http://www.healthline.com/health-blogs/fruit-womb/Asherman's-syndrome-diagnosis-treatment-and-prevention.
[30] Reddy, S; Rock, JA. Surgical management of complete obliteration of the endometrial cavity. *Fertil Steril*, 1997, 67, 172–174.
[31] Kodaman, PH; Arici, AA. "Intra-uterine adhesions and fertility outcome: how to optimize success?" *Current Opinion in Obstetrics and Gynecology*, 2007, 19 (3), 207–214.
[32] Valle, RF; Sciarra, JJ. Intrauterine adhesions: hysteroscopic diagnosis classification, treatment, and reproductive outcome. *Am J Obstet Gynecol*, 1988, 158, 1459–1470.
[33] Pabuccu, R; Atay, V; Orhon, E; Urman, B; Ergun, A. Hysteroscopic treatment of intrauterine adhesions is safe and effective in the restoration of normal menstruation and fertility. *Fertil Steril*, 1997, 68, 1141–1143.

[34] Shokeir, TA; Fawzy, M; Tatongy, M. The nature of intrauterine adhesions following reproductive hysteroscopic surgery as determined by early and late follow-up hysteroscopy: clinical implications. *Arch Gynecol Obstet*, 2008, 277, 423–427.

[35] Polishuk, WZ; Kohane, S. Intrauterine adhesions: diagnosis and therapy. *Obstet Gynecol Digest,* 1966, 8, 41.

[36] Ventolini, G; Zhang, M; Gruber, J. Hysteroscopy in the evaluation of patients with recurrent pregnancy loss. *Surg Endosc*, 2004, 18, 1782-1784.

[37] Vesce, F; Jorizzo, G; Bianciotto, A; Gotti, G. Use of the copper intrauterine device in the management of secondary amenorrhea. *Fertil Steril*, 2000, 73, 162-165.

[38] March, CM. Intrauterine adhesions. *Obstet Gynecol Clin North Am,* 1995, 22, 491-505.

[39] Tonguc, EA; Var, T; Yilmaz, N; Batioglu, S. Intrauterine device or estrogen treatment after hysteroscopic uterine septum resection. *Int J Gynaecol Obstet*, 2010, 109, 226-229.

[40] Deans, R; Abbott, J. Review of intrauterine adhesions**.** *J Minim Invasive Gynecol,* 2010, 17, 555-569.

[41] March, CM. Management of Asherman syndrome. *Reprod Biomed Online,* 2011, 23, 63-76.

[42] Lin, X; Wei, M; Li, TC; Huang, Q; Huang, D; Zhou, F; Zhang, S. A comparison of intrauterine balloon, intrauterine contraceptive device and hyaluronic acid gel in the prevention of adhesion reformation following hysteroscopic surgery for Asherman syndrome: a cohort study. *Eur J Obstet Gynecol Reprod Biol*, 2013, 170, 512-516.

[43] Amer, MI; Abd-El-Maeboud, KH. Amnion graft following hysteroscopic lysis of intrauterine adhesions. *J Obstet Gynaecol Res*, 2006, 32, 559-566.

[44] Orhue, AA; Aziken, ME; Igbefoh, JO. A comparison of two adjunctive treatments for intrauterine adhesions following lysis. *Int J Gynaecol Obstet*, 2003**,** 82, 49-56.

[45] Pellicano, M; Bramante, S; Cirillo, D; Palomba, S; Bifulco, G; Zullo, F; Nappi, C. Effectiveness of autocrosslinked hyaluronic acid gel after laparoscopic myomectomy in infertile patients: a prospective, randomized, controlled study. *Fertil Steril*, 2003, 80, 441-444.

[46] Guida, M; Acunzo, G; Di Spiezio Sardo, A; Bifulco, G; Piccoli, R; Pellicano, M; Cerrota, G; Cirillo, D; Nappi, C. Effectiveness of auto-crosslinked hyaluronic acid gel in the prevention of intrauterine adhesions after hysteroscopic surgery: a prospective, randomized, controlled study. *Hum Reprod,* 2004**,** 19, 1461-1464.

[47] Reijnen, MM; Falk, P; van Goor, H; Holmdahl, L. The antiadhesive agent sodium hyaluronate increases the proliferation rate of human peritoneal mesothelial cells. *Fertil Steril,* 2000, 74, 146-151.

[48] Mais, V; Cirronis, MG; Peiretti, M; Ferrucci, G; Cossu, E; Melis, GB. Efficacy of auto-crosslinked hyaluronan gel for adhesion prevention in laparoscopy and hysteroscopy: a systematic review and meta-analysis of randomized controlled trials. *Eur J Obstet Gynecol Reprod Biol*, 2012, 160, 1-5.

[49] Kim, T; Ahn, KH; Choi, DS; Hwang, KJ; Lee, BI; Jung, MH; Kim, JW; Kim, JH; Cha, SH; Lee, KH*;* et al. A randomized, multi-center, clinical trial to assess the efficacy and safety of alginate carboxymethylcellulosehyaluronic acid compared to carboxymethylcellulose hyaluronic acid to prevent postoperative intrauterine adhesion. *J Minim Invasive Gynecol*, 2012, 19, 731-736.

[50] Conforti, A; Alviggi, C; Mollo, A; Placido, GD; Magos, A. The management of Asherman syndrome: a review of literature. *Reproductive Biology and Endocrinology*, 2013, 11, 118 Available at: http://www.rbej.com/content/11/1/118.

[51] Sugimoto, O. Diagnostic and therapeutic hysteroscopy for traumatic intrauterine adhesions. *Am J Obstet Gynecol*, 1978, 131, 539-547.

[52] March, CM. Management of Asherman syndrome. *Reprod Biomed Online*, 2011, **23,** 63-76.

[53] Yu, D; Wong, YM; Cheong, Y; Xia, E; Li, TC. Asherman syndrome-one century later. *Fertil Steril*, 2008, 89, 759-779.

[54] Zinger, M; Liu, JH; Thomas, MA. Successful use of vaginal sildenafil citrate in two infertility patients with Asherman's syndrome. *J Womens Health (Larchmt)*, 2006, **15,** 442-444.

[55] Gargett, CE; Nguyen, HP; Ye, L. Endometrial regeneration and endometrial stem/progenitor cells. *Rev Endocr Metab Disord*, 2012, 13, 235-251.

[56] Nagori, CB; Panchal, SY; Patel, H. Endometrial regeneration using autologous adult stem cells followed by conception by *in vitro* fertilization in a patient of severe Asherman's syndrome. *J Hum Reprod Sci*, 2011, 4, 43-48.

[57] Kodaman, P; Arici, A. Intra-uterine adhesions and fertility outcome: how to optimize success? *Curr Opin Obstet Gynecol*, 2007, 19, 207-214.

In: Amenorrhea
Editor: Oliver Chukwujekwu Ezechi

ISBN: 978-1-63484-778-0

Chapter 12

SHEEHAN'S SYNDROME

Ayodeji A. Oluwole
Department of Obstetrics and Gynaecology, College of Medicine,
University of Lagos, Lagos University Teaching Hospital, Idi-Araba, Surulere, Lagos

SUMMARY

Sheehan's syndrome is postpartum hypopituitarism due to necrosis of the pituitary gland. This is as a result of severe hypovolaemia or shock from massive obstetric haemorrhage during or after delivery. The frequency is greatly reduced in developed countries because of improved obstetric services but same cannot be said in developing or under developed countries due to poor obstetric services and massive postpartum haemorrhage, which is also the greatest cause of morbidity and mortality in these countries. History of postpartum haemorrhage, cessation of menses and failure of lactation should greatly arouse suspicion. Early diagnosis and appropriate treatment will greatly reduce the adverse effects in women.

Keywords: Sheehan's syndrome, amenorrhea, pituitarism, obstetric haemorrhage

INTRODUCTION

Sheehan's syndrome (SS) is pituitary necrosis secondary to massive postpartum haemorrhage and hypovolaemia, with resulting partial or total pituitary hypofunction. It is mainly diagnosed retrospectively, sometimes after a delay of several years, as a classical cause of hypopituitarism. It was first described in 1937 by British pathologist, Harold L. Sheehan using observations of autopsy findings and symptoms of hypopituitarism in women that died from or survived massive postpartum haemorrhage.

Enlargement of pituitary gland, smaller sellar size, disseminated intravascular coagulation and autoimmunity have been suggested to play a role in the pathogenesis of Sheehan's syndrome. This syndrome is characterized by varying degrees of anterior pituitary dysfunction. Symptomatic posterior function is uncommon and many patients have impaired neurohypophyseal function tests. In many women with Sheehan's syndrome, anterior pituitary dysfunction remains undiagnosed for many years after the inciting delivery. The spectrum of clinical presentation ranges from non-specific complaints to severe pituitary insufficiency that may cause death. Advances in modern obstetric care have gradually decreased severe postpartum haemorrhage and Sheehan's syndrome all over the world, particularly in developed countries. The same may not be said in underdeveloped and developing countries, where majority of the deliveries are still poorly supervised and haemorrhage is still a leading cause of morbidity and mortality.

EPIDEMIOLOGY

Half a century ago, the prevalence was 10-20 per 100, 000 women. It is now uncommon, especially in developed countries, due to improvements in obstetric care. In the developing countries where home deliveries are widely practised and obstetric help is poor, Sheehan's syndrome is still a big health issue. The prevalence in India is estimated to be 2.7-3.9% among parous women older than 20years. In a retrospective analysis that was carried out in Iceland, the prevalence was estimated as 5.1 per 100, 000 women in 2009. In another study, the prevalence was found to be 3.1% in KIMS database of 1034 patients with growth hormone deficiency.

AETIOPATHOGENESIS

The vulnerability of the pituitary gland to damage during postpartum haemorrhage can be explained by its anatomy and blood supply as it is one of the most highly vascularised tissues in the body. Its volume increases two-fold in pregnancy, mostly due to the massive hyperplasia of lactotrophs as a result of elevated oestrogen secretion. The enlarged pituitary gland is vulnerable to ischemia and the gland does not have the ability to regenerate. Scar tissue replaces the necrotic cells. The necrotized area of the adenohypophysis undergo organization, form a fibrous scar leading to time-dependent atrophic changes of the pituitary gland resulting in empty sella turcica, the lodging bed of the pituitary gland. Infarction in the pituitary gland leads to replacement of functional cells by scar tissue and thus hypopituitarism (70-90% of gland affected). This is due to hypoperfusion from the massive blood loss; though vasospasm, thrombosis and vascular compression of the hypophyseal arteries have also been described as causes.

Factors thought to play a role in the pathogenesis include physiologic enlargement of pituitary gland in pregnancy, small sella size, disseminated intravascular coagulation and autoimmunity. The anterior pituitary is more commonly affected than the posterior. Pathogenesis of Sheehan's syndrome is proposed with some other factors. One of these factors is the size of the sella. Women with a sella smaller than average are expected to have a greater risk of Sheehan's syndrome. Sheehan's syndrome is characterized by slow progression of pituitary dysfunction several years after the last labour, and this suggests that other factors are involved in the pathogenesis of the disease. Some of these factors are anti-pituitary and anti-hypothalamic antibodies, which were shown to be present in some patients with Sheehan's syndrome, and this suggests that anti-immune pituitary process could be a causative factor.

Anti-pituitary antibodies, which can be detected in up to 63% of women with Sheehan's syndrome, can persist for years after the postpartum haemorrhage. Sequestered antigens due to tissue necrosis could trigger autoimmunity and may cause delayed hypopituitarism in these women. The antibodies may destroy remaining pituitary cells with time. Disseminated intravascular coagulation, which may worsen pituitary necrosis, can also occur in the context of postpartum anterior pituitary necrosis.

Clinical Presentation

The extent of pituitary dysfunction varies in women. In many affected women, anterior pituitary dysfunction is not diagnosed for many years. The main involvement is usually the secretion of growth hormone (GH) and prolactin (90-100%), while deficiencies in cortisol secretion, gonadotrophin and thyroid stimulating hormones (TSH) ranged from 50-100%. At least 75% of the pituitary must be destroyed before clinical manifestations become evident. Growth hormone deficiency is very common because somatrophs are located in the lower and lateral regions of the pituitary gland and are most likely to be damaged by ischemic necrosis of the pituitary. Neurohypophyseal functions have been shown to be frequently impaired in Sheehan's syndrome patients from the posterior pituitary dysfunction. Clinical diabetes insipidus is an uncommon complication of postpartum pituitary necrosis.

Haematological Abnormalities

Haematological abnormalities are also common and include those in Table 2 below:

Table 1. Clinical features of Sheehan's syndrome

History of postpartum haemorrhage
Lactation failure
Secondary amenorrhea
Breast atrophy
Decreased libido
Genital and axillary hair loss
Hypopigmentation
Premature ageing
Asthenia and weakness
Dry skin
Diabetes insipidus
Psychiatric disturbances, cognitive dysfunction
Changes in body composition
Hypotension and shock

Table 2. Haematological abnormalities in Sheehan's syndrome

Anaemia
Pancytopenia
Thrombocytopenia
Deranged PT and aPTT
High fibrinogen and d-dimer levels

Diagnosis

Diagnosis of Sheehan's syndrome is based on medical history, physical findings and evaluation of pituitary hormone levels. The most important issue in diagnosis is to be aware of the syndrome. Investigations include;

1. Hormone assay – prolactin, low Thyroid stimulating hormone, free T3, freeT4, Adrenocorticotrophic hormone (ACTH), Luteinising hormone (LH), Follicle stimulating hormone (FSH), cortisol, thyroxine, IGF-1 and estradiol.
2. Hormone stimulation tests include: insufficient responses of prolactin to Thyrotropin –releasing hormone (TRH), and GH to Insulin Tolerance test (ITT). Growth hormone (GH) deficiency is almost universal. Peak TSH response to TRH is insufficient, while baseline TSH level can be normal, low and even mildly elevated.
3. Radiology- computerised tomography (CT) or magnetic resonance imaging (MRI) of the brain. MRI will reveal enlarged non-haemorrhagic pituitary gland in early stages; the sella will be empty due to necrosis and atrophy in chronic stages. Size of empty sella may help in differential diagnosis of primary empty sella in Sheehan's syndrome. An empty sella has a normal size in Sheehan's syndrome and the pituitary fossa is large in primary empty sella syndrome.

Differential Diagnosis

Pituitary apoplexy, lymphocytic hypophysitis and primary empty sella syndrome should be uppermost on the mind. Hypopituitarism and pituitary gland enlargement can be observed in early stages of apoplexy occurring due to pituitary adenoma and early phases of Sheehan's syndrome. Lymphocytic hypophysitis is seen frequently in the postpartum period, and empty sella may develop as a result of the atrophy of pituitary gland in the long term. Also primary empty sella has similar findings in both diseases, having a large pituitary fossa without hypopituitarism may help differentiating from these diseases.

Treatment

The aim of treatment of Sheehan's syndrome is replacing the lack of hormones thereby improving the endocrinological disorder and reducing morbidity and mortality from hypopituitarism. The management should involve the endocrinologist.

Glucocorticoid replacement (hydrocortisone 20mg daily) is usually commenced before thyroid hormone replacement (thyroxine, titrated dose) to avoid a possible adrenal crisis. The dose should be higher in the morning and lower in the evening. By so doing, diurnal rhythm should be mimicked. These patients receiving steroid replacement should be evaluated for side effects including weight gain, glucose intolerance and bone mineral density.

Levothyroxine treatment should be administered to the patients having thyrotropin deficiency. Higher doses can be used in younger women and lower doses in older women. The aim is to maintain T4 level in the upper half of the normal range.

Oestrogen replacement, with or without progesterone is also indicated especially when osteoporosis develops in premenopausal women. Growth hormone treatment has a positive effect on the quality of life, body composition and lipid profile in these patients. Growth hormone treatment improves cognitive functions. Ovulation induction and hormonal supplementation for pregnancy is also an option for patients who may want to become pregnant.

Diabetes insipidus is typically managed with desmopressin (DDAVP).

CONCLUSION

Sheehan's syndrome is more common in developing countries due to poorer obstetric services. A high index of suspicion is required to suspect diagnosis as symptoms may be subtle and patients typically present years after the initial postpartum haemorrhage. History of postpartum haemorrhage, failure to lactate and cessation of menses are important clues to the diagnosis. Early diagnosis and prompt treatment are necessary to reduce morbidity and mortality in these patients.

REFERENCES

Abs, R; Bengtsson, BA; Hernberg-Stahl, E; et al. GH replacement in 1034 growth hormone deficiency hypopituitary adults: demographic and clinical characteristics, dosing and safety. *Clin Endocrinol (Oxf)*, 1999, 50, 703-13.

Cook, DM; Ludlam, WH; Cook, MB. Route of estrogen administration helps to determine growth hormone (GH) replacement dose in GH-deficient adults. *J Clin Endocrinol Metab*, 1999, 84, 3956-60.

De Bellis, A; Kelestimur, F; Sinisi, AA; et al. Anti-hypothalamus and anti-pituitary antibodies may contribute to perpetuate the hypopituitarism in patients with Sheehan's syndrome. *Eur J Endocrinol*, 2008, 158, 147-52.

Gei-Guardia, O; Soto-Herrera, E; Gei-Breasley, A; Chen-Ku, CH. Sheehan's Syndrome in Costa Rica. Clinical experience on 60 cases. *Endocr Pract*, 2010, 1, 1-27.

Gokalp, D; Tuzcu, A; Bahceci, M; et al. Assessment of bleeding disorders in Sheehan's syndrome; are bleeding disorders the underlying cause of Sheehan's syndrome? *Platelets*, 2011, 22, 92-7.

Goswami, R; Kochupillai, N; Crock, PA; et al. Pituitary autoimmunity in patients with Sheehan's syndrome. *J Clin Endocrinol Metab*, 2002, 87, 4137-41.

Karaca, Z; Tanriverdi, F; Unluhizarci, K; et al. Empty sella may be the final outcome in lymphocytic hypophysitis. *Endocr Res*, 2009, 34, 10-17.

Kristjansdottir, HL; Bodvarsdottir, SP; Sigurjonsdottir, HA. Sheehan's syndrome in modern times: a nationwide retrospective study in Iceland. *Eur J Endocrinol*, 2011, 164, 349-54.

Otsuka, F; Kageyama, J; Ogura, T; Hattori, T; Makino, H. Sheehan's syndrome of more than 30 years duration: An endocrine and MRI study of 6 cases. *Endocr J*, 1998, 45, 451-8.

Sheehan, HL. Postpartum necrosis of the anterior pituitary. *J Pathol bacterial*, 1937, 45, 189-214.

Sheehan, HL. The frequency of post partum hypopituitarism. *J Obstet Gynaecol Br Commonwealth*, 1965, 72, 103-111.

Sherif, IH; Vanderley, CM; Beshyah, S; et al. Sella size and contents in Sheehan's syndrome. *Clin Endocrinol (Oxf)*, 1989, 30, 613-8.

Shivaprasad, C. Sheehan's syndrome: Newer advances, *Indian J Endocr Metab*, 2011, 15, 203-7.

Takahiro, M; Khaleque, NK; Tsuneo, I; Atsushi, Y; Hideaki, M. Evaluation of obstetrical factors related to Sheehan's syndrome. *J Obstet Gynaecol Res*, 2014, 40, 46-52.

Tessnow, AH; Wilson, JD. The changing face of Sheehan's syndrome. *Am J Med Sci*, 2010, 340, 402-6.

Toogood, AA; Stewart, PM. Hypopituitarism: clinical features, diagnosis and management. *Endocrinol Metab Clin North Am*, 2008, 37, 235-61.

Yamauchi, T; Yoshio, N; Mizuguchi, T; et al. Acute fatty liver of pregnancy complicated with anterior pituitary insufficiency. *Intern Med*, 2001, 40, 1227-31.

In: Amenorrhea
Editor: Oliver Chukwujekwu Ezechi

ISBN: 978-1-63484-778-0

Chapter 13

HYPERPROLACTINAEMIA

Preye Owen Fiebai and Ngozi Clare Orazulike
Department of Obstetrics and Gynaecology, Faculty of Clinical Sciences,
College of Health Sciences, University of Port Harcourt, Port Harcourt, Nigeria

ABSTRACT

Hyperprolactinaemia is the most common endocrine disorder of the hypothalamic-pituitary-ovarian-axis. Elevated levels of serum prolactin (PRL) may result from physiological conditions, may be drug induced or may be pathologic. The prevalence of hyperprolactinaemia varies depending on the study population, but is reportedly higher in infertile women. Hyperprolactinaemia is thought to suppress gonadal function in several ways. It inhibits the positive estrogen feedback on luteinizing hormone (LH) secretion in women at the pituitary level. It also increases adrenal androgen secretion, and blocks the effects of gonadotropins at the gonadal level. Symptoms in women with hyperprolactinaemia may result from the effects of increased levels of PRL, from the effects of lesions causing the disorder, or from dysfunction of secretion of other anterior pituitary hormones. This may result in anovulation and presents as oligomenorrhoea or amenorrhea in women. Identification of the cause of hyperprolactinaemia is necessary for proper treatment. Patients may present with pituitary adenomas, which may or may not be radiologically detectable. Macroprolactinaemia and hook effect are challenges in laboratory diagnosis. Treatment with dopamine agonists is effective in over 80% of affected women with carbegoline being more effective and better tolerated than bromocriptine. Trans-sphenoidal hypophysectomy has a place in treatment of macroprolactinomas resistant to medical treatment and may be considered. Accurate diagnosis is critical to managing oligomenorrhoea/amenorrhea resulting from hyperprolactinaemia.

Keywords: hyperprolactinaemia, amenorrhea, prolactin, bromocriptine

INTRODUCTION

Prolactin (PRL) is a 198-amino acid peptide hormone mainly synthesized and secreted by the lactotroph cells of the anterior pituitary gland [1, 2]. Recent evidence suggests that extrapituitary production occurs and sites include the mammary gland, uterus, placenta and T lymphocytes [3, 4]. PRL has a molecular weight of 23kDa and its chemical structure is similar to growth hormone (GH) and human placental lactogen (HPL). These hormones also share genomic and biological activity, belonging to the same PRL/GH/HPL protein family [5]. There are three types of PRL – Little PRL, Big PRL and Big big PRL. Structural modifications resulting from glycosylation, phosphorylation, additions and deletions account for the different sizes and types of PRL. Little PRL has more bioactivity and immunoactivity than the other forms. In humans, PRL is encoded by a gene located on chromosome 6 [5-8].

PRL has a wide range of effects in human species and is best known for its role in the regulation of lactation [9-11]. Its primary function is the stimulation of breast epithelial cell proliferation and lactation. It has also been recently found to be involved in other biological activity including angiogenesis, osmoregulation and immunogenicity. This chapter focuses on the effect of excessive production of PRL on human reproduction with emphasis on oligomenorrhoea and infertility [9 -11].

BIOLOGICAL ACTION OF PROLACTIN

PRL's main biological function is induction and maintenance of lactation and any elevation of serum PRL levels outside pregnancy and the puerperium is abnormal [10, 11]. It acts on oestrogen and progesterone primed mammary glands to stimulate lactation. The high levels of oestrogen and progesterone inhibit lactation during pregnancy until the puerperium when these levels decline. Prolactin levels are high in the postpartum period and these high prolactin levels suppress ovulation during lactation and breastfeeding.

PATHOGENESIS

Hyperprolactinaemia is thought to suppress gonadal function in several ways. It inhibits the positive oestrogen feedback on luteinizing hormone (LH) secretion in women at the pituitary level. It also increases adrenal androgen secretion, and blocks the effects of gonadotropins at the gonadal level.

PRL secretion is under dual regulation by hypothalamic hormones. Unlike other pituitary hormones, PRL secretion is controlled primarily by inhibition via the neurotransmitter dopamine released from neurons in the hypothalamus into the portal system. Dopamine acts via D2 receptors on lactotrophs to tonically inhibit secretion of PRL. Gamma amino butyric acid (GABA), somatostatin, acetylcholine, and norepinephrine also inhibit prolactin release [12-17].

Stimulatory signals for PRL release are provided by the hypothalamic peptides, thyrotropin releasing hormone (TRH), vasoactive intestinal peptide (VIP), epidermal growth factor (EGF), and dopamine receptor antagonists [10, 11]. Nocturnal surges and suckling-induced prolactin rises are mediated by serotonin, which also modulates prolactin secretion. Histamine acts by inhibition of the dopaminergic system to stimulate PRL release [9-14].

Table 1. Aetiology of Hyperprolactinemia

Physiologic	Pathologic

Pregnancy
Lactation
Sleep
Stress
Chest wall stimulation
	Hypothalamic-pituitary stalk damage
	• Tumors
	  • Prolactinoma
	  • Craniopharyngioma
	  • Suprasellar pituitary mass
	  • Meningioma
	  • Dysgerminoma
	  • Metastatic tumours
	• Empty sella
	• Lymphocytic hypophysitis
	• Adenoma with stalk compression
	• Granulomas
	• Rathke's cyst
	• Irradiation
	• Trauma
	  • Pituitary stalk section
	  • Suprasellar surgery
	Systemic disorders
	• Chronic renal failure
	• Hypothyroidism
	• Cirrhosis
	• Pseudocyesis
	• Epileptic seizures
	• Acromegaly
	Dopamine receptor blockers
	• Atypical antipsychotics: risperidone
	• Phenothiazines: chlorpromazine, perphenazine
	• Butyrophenones: haloperidol
	• Thioxanthenes
	• Metoclopramide
	Dopamine synthesis inhibitors
	• α-Methyldopa
	Catecholamine depletors
	• Reserpine
	Opiates
	H2 antagonists
	• Cimetidine, ranitidine
	Imipramines
	• Amitriptyline, amoxapine
	Serotonin reuptake inhibitors
	• Fluoxetine
	Calcium channel blockers
	• Verapamil
	Estrogens
	TRH

PRL self regulates its secretion through the hypopyhseal pituitary portal system by a counter-current flow that causes secretion of dopamine from the hypothalamus and inhibition of gonadotropin releasing hormone (GnRH). This results in a reduction in secretion of pituitary hormones responsible for reproduction. The negative effect on the secretion of LH and follicle stimulating hormone (FSH) results in hypogonadotropic hypogonadism, anovulation and oligomenorrhoea/amenorrhea. The positive feedback of oestrogen on the release of LH at the pituitary level is inhibited by this action [14-18].

PRL is also believed to act directly on the ovary probably influencing ovarian steroidogenesis by its action on the aromatase enzyme [16]. In the follicular phase of the ovarian cycle, elevated PRL can disrupt normal follicular development and inhibit ovulation. Serum prolactin level is the result of a complex balance between positive and negative stimuli derived from both external and endogenous environments.

Hyperprolactinaemia is the most common endocrine disorder of the hypothalamic-pituitary-ovarian axis defined as an elevation of serum prolactin above a reference laboratory's upper limits [12, 15, 17-19]. A serum prolactin level of 500mIU/L (20ng/ml or μg/ml) or less is considered to be normal in women. Hyperprolactinaemia could be physiological, drug induced or pathological. The more common causes are idiopathic hyperprolactinaemia and lactotroph adenoma (prolactinoma). The aetiology of hyperprolactinaemia is summarized in Table 1.

Majority of cases of hyperprolactinaemia are caused by prolactinomas, which are benign tumours of the lactotroph cells of the anterior pituitary. They are classified according to their size into microadenomas (<10 mm) and macroadenomas (>10 mm) [17-20].

EPIDEMIOLOGY

The prevalence of hyperprolactinaemia varies depending on the study population. The actual prevalence of hyperprolactinaemia is difficult to determine because not all affected individuals are symptomatic or concerned with their symptoms while many are ignorant of the condition. A low prevalence of hyperprolactinaemia has been reported among healthy premenopausal women while high prevalence rates are reported amongst infertile women and women with galactorrhoea and menstrual disorders [21, 22]. Age prevalence varies widely and hyperprolactinaemia has been reported in prepubertal females and after the menopause [22].

Prevalence rates ranging from 0.4% in a healthy population to 9% among symptomatic women have been reported. High prevalence of 25% among women with galactorrhoea and 70% among those with galactorrhoea and amenorrhea have been documented [21-25].

CLINICAL FEATURES

The clinical features of hyperprolactinaemia may result from the direct effect of prolactin excess, from the effects of the cause of prolactin excess or from the resultant hypogonadotropic hypogonadism. The clinical presentation varies dependent on the age and the sex of the patient and the magnitude of hyperprolactinaemia [10-12, 15, 17, 18].

It is important to take a detailed history from the patient to exclude causes of hyperprolactinaemia such as drugs, chest wall trauma/surgery and systemic diseases. Affected women usually present with a history of galactorrhoea, infertility, oligomenorrhoea, amenorrhea or decreased libido [24-28].

Patients who have macroadenomas could present with neurological symptoms caused by mass effects of the tumor. Symptoms include headaches, visual field impairment, cranial neuropathies, hypopituitarism, seizures, and cerebrospinal fluid rhinorrhea [29].

The incidence of galactorrhoea amongst women with hyperprolactinaemia is variable and ranges between 20 – 90% [27]. When galactorrhoea occurs in women with amenorrhea/oligomenorrhoea it is likely to be associated with hyperprolactinaemia but when it occurs in women with normal menstrual cycles, hyperprolactinaemia is unlikely. Many premenopausal women with hyperprolactinaemia do not present with galactorrhoea and galactorrhoea may occur with normal prolactin levels [26, 27].

Infertility may result from the effects of hyperprolactinaemia on the reproductive process through interference with the hypothalamic-pituitary-ovarian axis or through a direct effect on the ovaries. Hyperprolactinaemia inhibits the release of GnRH from the hypothalamus. This affects the release of the pituitary gonadotrophins (FSH and LH), resulting in hypogonadotrophic hypogonadism characterized by anovulation and menstrual disorders.

Menstrual irregularities ranging from oligomenorrhoea to amenorrhea may also occur. The pattern is variable but markedly elevated PRL levels are associated with anovulation and amenorrhea. Mild hyperprolactinaemia may not present with amenorrhea but marked elevation of PRL commonly presents with amenorrhea. Elevated PRL can also disrupt normal follicular development in the follicular phase, cause atresia of the dominant follicle and anovulation.

Physical examination of women with hyperprolactinaemia may reveal no other feature than galactorrhoea. Other physical signs if present could reflect the cause of hyperprolactinaemia, the most common cause being a pituitary adenoma. Microadenomas do not usually manifest with physical signs but macroadenomas may compress the optic chiasma resulting in visual impairment. Examination of the visual fields is therefore necessary to exclude optic nerve compression, which usually presents with bi-temporal hemianopsia.

INVESTIGATION

Laboratory Investigations

Definitive diagnosis of hyperprolactinaemia can only be made with laboratory investigations. A serum prolactin level above 20 μg/L is indicative of hyperprolactinaemia but cannot determine the cause. The aim of evaluation should be to distinguish between pathologic and physiologic hyperprolactinaemia. Serum PRL levels between 20 - 200μg/L may be associated with secondary causes of hyperprolactinaemia but levels above 200 μg/L usually indicate the presence of a prolactinoma [30, 31].

Before collection of blood samples for prolactin assay, the patient should be fasted for 8 to 10 hours and should not have engaged in rigorous exercise [32]. The sample should be taken in the morning at least 2 hours after sleep and ideally without a tourniquet.

A single mild elevation in serum prolactin should be re-evaluated and the levels should be markedly elevated before labeling the patient as hyperprolactinaemic. Macroprolactinaemia and ‘hook effect’ are challenges in laboratory diagnosis.

Human prolactin circulates in monomeric and polymeric forms, which are indistinguishable by routine assays. Macroprolactinaemia results from binding of prolactin to IgG antibodies creating a polymeric form of prolactin, which is detected by the usual immunological assay methods. The large polymer is unable to bind with the prolactin receptor and has little or no biological activity. Precipitation with polyethylene glycol is useful in detection of macroprolactinaemia, which is a significant cause of misdiagnosis and unnecessary treatment [19, 31].

Giant macroprolactinomas on the other hand may be associated with very high levels of serum prolactin, which may be underestimated due to the so-called 'hook effect.' Saturation of both capture and signal antibodies of two-site immunometric assays by large amounts of PRL impairs binding causing underestimation of their levels [19, 31].

Imaging Studies

When hyperprolactinaemia is confirmed, imaging of the pituitary fossa preferably by magnetic resonance imaging (MRI) is recommended to determine the presence of a prolactinoma or any other hypothalamic/pituitary lesion. Computed tomography (CT) is not as sensitive as MRI in the detection of small pituitary lesions [19, 22, 6, 31, 32].

TREATMENT

The treatment of hyperprolactinaemia depends on the underlying aetiology. Affected patients can be categorized into 3 groups with respect to treatment (Table 2).

Group 1

Medical therapy with dopamine agonists that have been in clinical use for many years is the mainstay of management in this category of patients. They have been proven to be very effective in normalizing serum prolactin levels, reversing amenorrhea/oligomenorrhoea and restoring ovulation and fertility.

Most commonly used dopamine agonists are bromocriptine and cabergoline. Others include lisuride, pergolide, quinagolide, terguride, and metergoline. With the exception of quinagolide, all these dopamine agonists are ergot alkaloids. Side effects are common especially with bromocriptine and include nausea, vomiting, headache, constipation, dizziness, faintness, depression, postural hypotension, digital vasospasm, and nasal stuffiness. Symptoms are more pronounced on commencement of the drug or with dose increment. Auditory hallucination, delusion and mood changes are rare side effects. Side effects usually resolve with discontinuation of the drugs [34-6].

Table 2. Categorization of Hyperprolactinemia patient based on required treatment

Group 1	Idiopathic or microadenoma associated hyperprolactinaemia	Medical management
Group 2	Hyperprolactinoma with macroadenoma	Medical management and surgery/radiotherapy
Group 3	Miscellaneous resulting from drugs, systemic disorders, stalk compression	Treatment of underlying cause

Bromocriptine is the first choice drug in this category and has been utilized for the longest period of time. It is a lysergic acid derivative with a bromine substitute at position 2 [37]. It is a strong dopamine agonist which binds to dopamine receptor and directly inhibits PRL secretion. It decreases prolactin synthesis, DNA synthesis, cell multiplication, and overall size of prolactinoma. It has a short half-life that necessitates twice daily administration to maintain serum levels.

It is best administered continuously and treatment is usually initiated at low doses and increased gradually by 1.25mg. Intolerance to bromocriptine is common and can be reduced by starting with the lowest dose of 1.25mg after supper with weekly increment by 1.25mg until serum PRL levels are normal. Therapeutic doses of bromocriptine range from 2.5mg to 15mg daily. Serum PRL levels usually reduce in about a week; ovulation and menstruation resumes in 4-8 weeks. Ovulatory function can be assessed by weekly serum progesterone assay in women with oligo - or amenorrhea. Alternative methods of administration include slow release oral form, and long acting intramuscular injection [37, 38]. Vaginal administration of bromocriptine is reported to allow lower therapeutic dosing as absorption is effective and the liver first pass metabolism is avoided [39]. Discontinuation of bromocriptine therapy is associated with return to elevated PRL levels in many patients. It is difficult to predict those patients in whom this will occur.

Cabergoline has similar characteristics and adverse effects with bromocriptine but has a very long half-life allowing weekly dosing. A weekly dose of 0.25mg to a maximum of 1.0mg is usually effective for hyperprolactinaemia. Doses as high as 4.5mg weekly have been used. It is more effective than bromocriptine in suppressing PRL and reducing tumour size [40, 41]. It can also be administered vaginally if poorly tolerated when taken orally [42].

Idiopathic Hyperprolactinemia

Bromocriptine is usually effective first line treatment in women with idiopathic hyperprolactinaemia. Continuous therapy results in reduction of serum PRL levels in a short period of time. Women with oligomenorrhoea or amenorrhea resume ovulation in 4 – 8 weeks if primarily caused by hyperprolactinaemia. Therapy is monitored with serum PRL and progesterone assays. Gonadotropin stimulation may be needed alongside dopamine agonist therapy to achieve ovulation in some patients.

Microadenoma with Hyperprolactinemia

Medical management with dopamine agonists usually lasts longer in this group of patients. Treatment can extend for periods ranging from 6 months to 6 years. No treatment is required in asymptomatic patients and those with very slowly growing tumours. Annual evaluation of prolactin levels, visual fields and tumour size by MRI is mandatory for follow-up. Oestrogen deficit should be replenished by hormone replacement therapy in amenorrhoiec women.

Group 2

Treatment in this group of patients is aimed at correcting the effects of hyperprolactinaemia including restoration of fertility, suppression of galactorrhea, prevention of bone loss and reduction of tumour mass. Response to therapy is variable and dopamine agonists are the first line of treatment. Shrinkage of macroprolactinomas is rapid in some cases while in others prolonged therapy may be required [44, 45]. Surgery and radiotherapy may be necessary in patients who are intolerant of, or who do not respond to medical therapy. Trans-sphenoidal, transnasal and transcranial surgery have been applied with different cure rates. Morbidity and mortality rates associated with surgery are high especially with giant pituitary adenomas. Postoperative persistence of hyperprolactinaemia and tumour residue are further challenges encountered after surgery. Hypopituitarism is also a long-term effect and should be discussed with the patient before surgery. Radiotherapy is reserved for patients with residual tumour after surgery. Dopamine agonists are still useful in managing patients with residual hyperprolactinaemia after surgery and radiotherapy.

Group 3

Treatment of hyperprolactinaemia resulting from systemic disease or drugs should take consideration of the patients health. Withdrawal of drugs should be carried out if the benefits outweigh the risks. Treatment of hypothyroidism and chronic renal failure usually result in correction of mild hyperprolactinaemia associated with these conditions.

Hyperprolactinaemia in Pregnancy

Dopamine agonists have been used safely in the first trimester of pregnancy without increased adverse effects on the fetus or the mother. There is a tendency to stop drug therapy in patients who are anovulatory and conceive during treatment. Increased growth of pituitary adenomas is not uncommon and dopamine agonists may need to be recommenced. There has been more experience with the use of bromocriptine than with carbegoline and other drugs but no significant adverse effects have been reported with both drugs [46].

Conclusion

The diagnosis of hyperprolactinaemia needs to be confirmed before treatment is commenced and dopamine agonists are the mainstay of treatment. Carbegoline is more effective than bromocriptine in achieving normal serum prolactin levels, and reestablishing ovulation and menstruation in women with oligomenorrhoea and amenorrhea. Surgery and radiotherapy may be needed in patients intolerant to dopamine agonist treatment or in those who do not respond to treatment.

REFERENCES

[1] Riddle, O; Bates, RW; Dykshorn, SW. The preparation, identification and assay of prolactin- a hormone of the anterior pituitary. *Am J Physiol.*, 1993, 105, 191.

[2] Freeman, ME; Kanyicska, B; Lerant, A; Nagy, G. Prolactin: structure, function, and regulation of secretion. *Physiological Reviews*, 2000, 80, 1523–1631.

[3] Ben Jonathan, N; Mershon, JL; Allen, DL; Steinmetz, RW. Extrapituitary prolactin distribution, regulation, functions, and clinical aspects. *Endocr Rev.*, 1996, 17, 639–669.

[4] Gerlo, S; Davis, JR; Mager, DL; Kooijman, R. "Prolactin in man: a tale of two promoters." *BioEssays*, 28, (10), 1051–5.

[5] Horseman, ND; Yu-Lee, LY. Transcriptional regulation by the helix bundle peptide hormones: growth hormone, prolactin, and hematopoietic cytokines. *Endocrine Review*, 1994, 15, 627–649.

[6] Suh, HK; Frantz, AG. Size heterogeneity of human prolactin in plasma and pituitary extracts. *J Clin Endocrinol Metab.*, 1974, 39(5), 928-35.

[7] Sinha, YN. Structural variants of prolactin: occurrence and physiological significance. *Endocr Rev.*, 1995, 16(3), 354-69.

[8] Jackson, RD; Wortsman, J; Malarkey, WB. Characterization of a large molecular weight prolactin in women with idiopathic hyperprolactinemia and normal menses. *J Clin Endocrinol Metab.*, 1985, 61(2), 258-64.

[9] Anne Bachelot and Nadine Binart. Reproductive role of prolactin. *Reproduction*, 2007,133, (2) 361-369.

[10] Bronstein, MD. Disorders of prolactin secretion and prolactinomas. In: DeGroot LJ, Jameson JL, editors. Endocrinology. *6th ed.* Philadelphia: Saunders/Elsevier, 2010, 333-57.

[11] Melmed, S; Casanueva, FF; Hoffman, AR; Kleinberg, DL; Montori; VM; Schlechte, JA; et al. Diagnosis and treatment of hyperprolactinemia: An Endocrine Society clinical practice guideline. *J Clin Endocrinol Metab.*, 2011, 96(2), 273-88.

[12] Majumdar, A; Mangal, NS. Hyperprolactinaemia. *J Hum Reprod Sci.*, 2013, 6(3), 168–175.

[13] Brooks, CL. Molecular mechanisms of prolactin and its receptor. *Endocrine Reviews*, 2012, 33, 504–525.

[14] Freeman, ME; Kanyicska, B; Lerant, A; Nagy, G. Prolactin: Structure, function, and regulation of secretion. *Physiol Rev.*, 2000, 80, 1523–631.

[15] Chahal, J; Schlechte, J. Hyperprolactinemia. *Pituitary.*, 2008, 11, 141–6.

[16] Martikainen, H; Rönnberg, L; Puistola, U; Tapanainen, J; Orava, M; Kauppila, A. Prolactin suppression by bromocriptine stimulates aromatization of testosterone to estradiol in women. *Fertil Steril.*, 1989, 52(1), 51-4.

[17] Mah, PM; Webster, J. Hyperprolactinemia: etiology, diagnosis, and management. *Semin Reprod Med.*, 2002, 20(4), 365-74.

[18] Abha, Majumdar; Nisha, Sharma Mangal. Hyperprolactinemia. *J Hum Reprod Sci.*, 2013, 6(3), 168–175.

[19] Vilar, Lucio; Fleseriu, Maria; Bronstein Marcello, D. Challenges and pitfalls in the diagnosis of hyperprolactinemia. *Arq Bras Endocrinol Metab.*, 2014, 58(1), 9-22.

[20] Glezer, Andrea; Bronstein, Marcello D. Prolactinoma. *Arq Bras Endocrinol Metab.*, 2014, 58(2), 118-123.

[21] Alpañés, M; Sanchón, R; Martínez-García, MÁ; Martínez-Bermejo, E; Escobar-Morreale, HF. Prevalence of hyperprolactinaemia in female premenopausal blood donors. *Clin Endocrinol (Oxf).*, 2013, 79(4), 545-9.

[22] Josimovich, JB; Lavenhar, MA; Devanesan, MM; Sesta, HJ; Wilchins SA; Smith, AC. Heterogeneous distribution of serum prolactin values in apparently healthy young women, and the effects of oral contraceptive medication. *Fertil Steril*, 1987, 47, 785-91.

[23] Bassey, IE; Udoh AE; Essien, OE; Isong, IK; Gali, RM; Archibong, EE. Thyroid hormones and prolactin levels in infertile women in southern Nigeria. *J Clin Diagn Res.*, 2015, 9(3), OC13-5.

[24] Luciano, AA. Clinical presentation of hyperprolactinemia. *J Reprod Med.*, 1999, 44(Suppl 12), 1085–90.

[25] Lee, DY; Oh, YK; Yoon, BK; Choi, D. Prevalence of hyperprolactinemia in adolescents and young women with menstruation-related problems. *Am J Obstet Gynecol.*, 2012, 206, 213.e1-5.

[26] Crosignani, PG. Current treatment issues in female hyperprolactinaemia. *Eur J Obstet Gynecol Reprod Biol.*, 2006, 125(2), 152-64.

[27] Huang, W; Molitch, ME. Evaluation and management of galactorrhea. *Am Fam Physician.*, 2012, 85(11), 1073-80.

[28] Webster, J, Scanlon, MF. Prolactinomas. In: Sheaves R, Jenkins PJ, Wass JA, editors. Clinical Endocrine Oncology. *Oxford: Blackwell Science*, 1997, 189–94.

[29] Lake, MG1; Krook, LS; Cruz, SV. Pituitary adenomas: an overview. *Am Fam Physician.*, 2013, 88(5), 319-27.

[30] Gibney, J; Smith, TP; McKenna, TJ. The impact on clinical practice of routine screening for macroprolactin. *J Clin Endocrinol Metab.*, 2005, 90, 3927–32.

[31] Omar, Serri; Constance, L. Chik; Ehud, Ur; Shereen, Ezzat. Diagnosis and management of hyperprolactinemia. *CMAJ*, 2003, 169(6), 575-81.

[32] Rao, Ar; Rao, KA. Hyperprolactinaemia and thyroid disorders. In Rao K, Carp H, editors, The Infertility Manual, 3rd ed. New Delhi, Jaypee Brothers Medical Publishers (P) Ltd, 2009, 95 – 101.

[33] Melmed, S; Casanueva, FF; Hoffman, AR; Kleinberg, DL; Montori, VM; Schlechte, JA; et al. Endocrine Society. Diagnosis and treatment of hyperprolactinemia: An endocrine society clinical practice guideline. *J Clin Endocrinol Metab.*, 2011, 96, 273–88.

[34] Schlechte, JA. Long-term management of prolactinomas. *J Clin Endocrinol Metab.*, 2007, 92, 2861–5.

[35] Turner, TH; Cookson, JC; Wass, JA; Drury, PL; Price, PA; Besser, GM. Psychotic reactions during treatment of pituitary tumours with dopamine agonists. *Br Med J (Clin Res Ed)*, 1984, 289, 1101–3.

[36] Motazedian, S; Babakhani, L; Fereshtehnejad, SM; Mojthahedi, K. A comparison of bromocriptine and cabergoline on fertility outcome of hyperprolactinemic infertile women undergoing intrauterine insemination. *Indian J Med Res.*, 2010, 131, 670–4.

[37] Merola, B; Colao, A; Caruso, E; Sarnacchiaro, F; Briganti, F; Lancranjan, I; et al. Oral and injectable longlasting bromocriptine preparations in hyperprolactinemia:

Comparison of their prolactin lowering activity, tolerability and safety. *Gynecol Endocrinol.*, 1991, 5, 267–76.
[38] Brue, T; Lancranjan, I; Louvet, JP; Dewailly, D; Roger, P; Jaquet, P. A long-acting repeatable form of bromocriptine as long-term treatment of prolactin-secreting macroadenomas: A multicenter study. *Fertil Steril.*, 1992, 57, 74–80.
[39] Katz, E; Weiss, BE; Hassell, A; Schran, HF; Adashi, EY. Increased circulating levels of bromocriptine after vaginal compared with oral administration. *Fertil Steril.*, 1991, 55, 882–4.
[40] Vance, ML; Evans, WS; Thorner, MO. Drugs five years later. Bromocriptine. *Ann Intern Med.*, 1984, 100, 78–91.
[41] Di Sarno, A; Landi, ML; Cappabianca, P; Di Salle, F; Rossi FW; Pivonello, R; et al. Resistance to cabergoline as compared with bromocriptine in hyperprolactinemia: Prevalence, clinical definition, and therapeutic strategy. *J Clin Endocrinol Metab.*, 2001, 86, 5256–61.
[42] Motta, T; de Vincentiis, S; Marchini, M; Colombo, N; D'Alberton, A. Vaginal cabergoline in the treatment of hyperprolactinemic patients intolerant to oral dopaminergics. *Fertil Steril.*, 1996, 65, 440–2.
[43] Gillam, MP; Molitch, ME; Lombardi, G; Colao, A. Advances in the treatment of prolactinomas. *Endocr Rev.*, 2006, 27, 485–534.
[44] Essaïs, O; Bouguerra, R; Hamzaoui, J; Marrakchi, Z; Hadjri, S; Chamakhi, S; et al. Efficacy and safety of bromocriptine in the treatment of macroprolactinomas. *Ann Endocrinol (Paris)*, 2002, 63, 524–31.
[45] Webster, J; Scanlon, MF. Prolactinomas. In: Sheaves R, Jenkins PJ, Wass JA, editors. Clinical Endocrine Oncology. *Oxford: Blackwell Science*, 1997. 189–94.
[46] Molitch, ME. Endocrinology in pregnancy: management of the pregnant patient with a prolactinoma. *Eur J Endocrinol.*, 2015, 172(5), R205-13.

In: Amenorrhea
Editor: Oliver Chukwujekwu Ezechi
ISBN: 978-1-63484-778-0

Chapter 14

PREMATURE OVARIAN FAILURE

Ngozi Clare Orazulike and Preye Owen Fiebai
Department of Obstetrics and Gynaecology, Faculty of Clinical Sciences,
College of Health Sciences, University of Port Harcourt, Port Harcourt, Nigeria

ABSTRACT

Premature ovarian failure (POF), also termed primary ovarian insufficiency is defined as the cessation of menses accompanied by raised gonadotrophin levels before the age of 40 years. The exact incidence of spontaneous POF is unknown as many are unrecognized; however, estimates vary between 1% and 5% of the female population. Currently, a rise in incidence of iatrogenic POF has been documented as many women are surviving cancers due to improved treatment modalities. Although most cases of POF are idiopathic, known causes include X-chromosome abnormalities and autosomal genetic conditions such as Turner's and Fragile X syndromes, autoimmune diseases, infections, iatrogenic agents that cause permanent damage to the ovaries. Menstrual irregularity including amenorrhea, hypo-estrogenism and elevated gonadotrophin levels characterize POF. Patients may present with infertility, and short and long term effects of estrogen deficiency. The diagnosis of POF is confirmed by two elevated FSH levels in the menopausal range (> 40IU/L) at least one month apart after 4 - 6 months of amenorrhea. Exogenous hormone replacement is necessary to restore normal menstrual cycles and decrease consequences of estrogen deficiency. Invitro fertilization with egg donation is recommended for women desiring child bearing. Life style modification and laparoscopic ovarian transposition before pelvic radiotherapy may prevent some cases of POF.

Keywords: premature ovarian failure, hormone, menopause, amenorrhea, menstrual irregularity

INTRODUCTION

Menopause occurs in 90% of women between the age of 45 and 55 years with the average age being 51 years [1, 2]. Premature ovarian failure (POF), which ultimately leads to premature menopause is defined as the cessation of menses before the age of 40 years [3]. It is associated with amenorrhea, sex steroid deficiency and elevated levels of serum gonadotropins before the age of 40 years typically as a result of loss of follicles, folliculogenesis and estrogen production. Amenorrhea is not essential for the diagnosis of POF as spontaneous menstrual cycles can occasionally occur after the diagnosis has been made.

Premature ovarian failure is also associated with physical and psychological consequences due to the symptoms and long-term effects of sex steroid deficiency as well as emotional sequelae experienced by couples desirous of childbearing, infertility being a devastating diagnosis.

It was Fuller Albright in 1942, considered by many to be the father of modern endocrinology that first reported on this newly recognized syndrome in young women. He called it, "primary ovarian insufficiency" (POI) to differentiate it from secondary ovarian insufficiency caused by a central defect in gonadotropin secretion by the pituitary [4]. Currently, 'primary ovarian insufficiency' or 'premature ovarian dysfunction' are terms increasingly being used and preferred to POF as they reflect the unpredictable nature of ovarian function in this condition which is a continuum rather than a specific end point [3, 5, 6]. POF which can be seen as the end point of POI is used in this book.

POF may occur at any age. The exact incidence is unknown as many go unrecognized. However, estimates vary between 1-2% of women younger than 40 years of age and 0.1% of women younger than 30 years of age [7]. It is estimated that 1 in 100 women will be affected by the condition by the age of 40 years while 1 in 10,000 women will be affected by 20 years of age [8].

The underlying etiologic mechanisms, natural history, medical and psychosocial management of POF are still poorly understood. Thus, the woman with POF requires integrated care for her physical, psychosocial, and reproductive health as well as preventive strategies to maintain her long-term fitness.

PATHOGENESIS

Most cases of premature ovarian failure are idiopathic, with no identifiable cause. However diverse etiologies have been found to be associated with POF: genetic aberrations, autoimmune ovarian damage, iatrogenic factors, and infectious agents (Table 1).

Table 1. Causative factors of premature ovarian failure

1. Idiopathic causes
2. Genetic disorders a. X chromosomal abnormalities b. X monosomy (Turner's syndrome) c. X Trisomy d. X- autosomal translocation e. X- chromosomal deletion f. Fragile X syndrome g. Mosaic karyotype h. Autosomal disorders

2. Genetic disorders (Continued) i. Galactosemia j. Steroidogenic enzyme defect k. Gonadotropin receptor dysfunction l. Inhibin gene mutation
C. Autoimmunologic causes **D. Iatrogenic causes** a. Pelvic surgery b. Irradiation c. Chemotherapy **E. Infectious Causes** a. Varicella b. Mumps c. Cytomegalovirus d. Tuberculosis e. Malaria f. Shigella **F. Environmental toxins**

Familial and Genetic Causes

Genetic disorders that involve the X chromosome or autosomes have been shown to be associated with development of POF. Available in the literature are list of newly discovered mutations that may be responsible for POF. Most of these mutations are extremely rare and thus most cases of POF are still considered to be idiopathic.

The genetic mechanisms implicated in the pathogenesis of POF include reduced gene dosage and non-specific chromosome effects that impair meiosis. These can cause a decrease in the pool of primordial follicles causing ovarian failure, apoptosis causing increased atresia of the follicles or failure of follicle maturation [9].

X Chromosomal Abnormalities

This could include a small defect in chromosomal arrangements such as deletions, isochromosomes and balanced X chromosome-autosomal translocations. They account for as much as 5% of cases [9]. Turner's syndrome characterized by a 45, XO karyotype is the most common chromosomal defect in humans [10]. Women with this syndrome characterized by primary amenorrhea, short stature and characteristic phenotypic features initially have a normal complement of ovarian follicles, which are rapidly lost before puberty. The identification of genes or critical regions responsible for individual Turner's syndrome has not been easy contrary to initial thoughts. However in POF patients, these deletions have been localized to chromosome Xq21.3-Xq27 (POF1) while balanced X/autosomal translocations have been localized to Xq13.3-q21.1 (POF2). The degrees of ovarian dysfunction and extent of somatic anomalies in Turner's syndrome are variable. While most affected patients have primary amenorrhea, streak gonads and absence of pubertal development, some especially the mosaic Turner's develop normally and occasionally have a successful pregnancy and then secondary amenorrhea while others have no somatic defects.

Autosomal Causes

These have been observed in patients with POF. An association between trisomy X and POF has been reported [11, 12]. POF has also been implicated in a girl with 48XXXX [13]; patients with Trisomy 18 and 13. Some autosomal genes have been implicated by autosome:autosome translocations although these are rare in POF. They include gene defects that cause the following autosomal disorders – Galactosemia, Blepharophimosis-ptosis-epicanthus inversus syndrome (BPES), Autoimmune polyendocrinopathy-candidiasis-ectodermal dystrophy (APECED), Steroidogenic enzyme defect, Gonadotropin receptor dysfunction, Inhibin gene mutation and Noggin mutation. These autosomal translocations may be chance findings appearing occasionally in women with POF without necessarily playing a significant causal role [14].

Fragile X Syndrome

This is the most common hereditary cause of mental retardation and developmental delay [15]. It is an X-linked dominant condition which is caused by an abnormality in the fragile X mental retardation 1 (*FMR1*) gene located on the X chromosome at Xq27.3. Women with full mutation have an average risk of developing POF while those with a pre-mutation have ten times higher the risk of developing POF [16].

There are examples of significant family histories of POF and it is estimated that 20 – 30% of cases of POF will have a family history identified [17]. This figure could be an over estimation due to inability to confirm family histories or an under estimation due to the fact that causative genes could be inherited through males and some women do not talk about the issue of POF with their families.

Auto Immune Causes

Abnormal self-recognition by the immune system may lead to some cases of POF. The exact causal mechanism remains poorly understood. Some of the evidence for auto immune aetiology includes the presence of lymphocytic oophoritis, demonstration of ovarian antibodies although their specificity and pathogenic role are obscure and associated autoimmune antibodies [18-20]. In 15%–20% of patients with POF, an autoimmune disease is also present [21]. Autoimmune POF can be seen as isolated or as part of autoimmune polyglandular diseases. More than 60% of these syndromes develop ovarian failure. Type 1 autoimmune polyglandular syndrome is rare, occurs at a young age and is autosomal recessively inherited. It causes hypoparathyroidism, mucocutaneous candidiasis, primary hypogonadism, and hypoadrenalism. Polyglandular autoimmune syndrome type 2 is more common, seen in adult patients, and has polygenic inheritance associated with HLA-DR3 and HLA-DR4. It causes adrenal insufficiency, autoimmune thyroid disease, type 1 diabetes, and gonadal failure. In patients with POF, other autoimmune diseases, such as vitiligo, myasthenia gravis, Sjögren's syndrome, systemic lupus erythematosus, celiac disease, rheumatoid arthritis, alopecia areata, Cushing's disease, Hashimoto's disease and pernicious anemia, may occur. In 11% of patients with POF, lymphocytic oophoritis is present, and steroid cell antibodies are present in 78% [22].

In POF due to autoimmune causes, the elevated serum gonadotropin hormones are due to dysfunction of the ovarian follicles rather than depletion. The primordial follicles are spared the lymphatic infiltration as only the secondary and antral follicles are affected. Thus resumption of ovarian function can occur with or without conception in a good number of affected individuals. (Table 2)

Table 2. Mechanism and etiology of premature ovary failure

Causative Factor	Mechanism	Type
Familial/Genetic	Reduced gene dosage and non-specific chromosome defects impair meiosis, which causes decreased pool of primordial follicles. Apoptosis causes increased atresia of follicles or failure of follicule maturation.	Turner's syndrome, Trisomy 13 and 18, Galactosemia, BPES, APECED, Inhibin gene mutation, Noggin mutation, Fragile X syndrome
Autoimmune	Dysfunction of ovarian follicles due to lymphatic infiltration.	Polyglandular autoimmune syndrome (Type 1 and 2), associated conditions such as Myasthenia gravis, Vitiligo, Hashimoto's disease, Cushing's syndrome, SLE, Pernicious anemia
Iatrogenic	Decrease in number of oocytes by damage to the DNA. Disrupts structure and function of oocyte and granulosa cells. Surgery disrupts blood supply to the ovaries.	Chemo- and radio-therapy, pelvic adnexal surgeries for Endometriosis or premenstrual syndrome, Uterine artery embolization
Infection	Inflammation and damage to oocytes.	Tuberculosis, Malaria, Varicella, Shigella, CMV, Mumps oophoritis, HIV
Environmental toxins	Disrupts function of oocytes	Smoking, Epilepsy

Iatrogenic Causes

Chemotherapy and radiation therapy for the treatment of malignant diseases are the most common causes of POF. Due to the improved success in treatment of cancer in children, adolescents and reproductive-age women and the practice of prophylactic bilateral oophorectomy at hysterectomy, the incidence of iatrogenic POF has increased over time. The effects of chemotherapy are age, dose- and drug-dependent, as well as concomitant radiotherapy. Alkylating agents such as cyclophosphamide are known to carry a much higher risk than vinca alkaloids, antimetabolites and anthracycline antibiotics. Chemotherapy reduces the number of oocytes by damaging the DNA and disrupts the structure and function of the oocyte and granulosa cells. Premature ovarian failure due to chemotherapeutics may be temporary; however, spontaneous recovery of ovarian function is less likely in older patients. In order to reducc the gonadotoxic effects of chemotherapy, simultaneous provision of GnRH analogs may be helpful [23].

Radiotherapy affects the ovaries, depending on the radiation area, dose of radiation and age of the individual. Prepubertal ovaries are relatively more resistant to radiation [24]. Laparoscopic ovarian transposition before pelvic radiation therapy helps to preserve ovarian function and thus reduce the risk of POF [25]. Studies have reported spontaneous return of ovarian function after several years in women with chemotherapy- or radiotherapy-induced ovarian failure and successful pregnancies even reported amongst them [26, 27] although the pregnancies may be complicated by increased miscarriage rates, small for gestational age (SGA) offspring and reduction in live births [28]. Younger age at first chemotherapy and absence of concomitant radiotherapy are predictive factors for spontaneous ovarian recovery.

Pelvic adnexal surgeries especially for benign gynaecological disorders such as endometriosis or premenstrual syndrome have the potential to damage the ovaries and cause POF by disrupting the ovarian blood supply and causing inflammation in the pelvic area. If sufficient collateral circulation develops, ovarian function may resume. Uterine artery embolization can also result in POF via compromise of ovarian blood supply.

Infectious Causes

Infections such as pelvic tuberculosis, malaria, varicella, shigella, cytomegalovirus and herpes simplex have been associated with POF [29]. Mumps oophoritis has also been implicated [30, 9]. In these patients, mainly menstrual cycle disorders and infertility occur. Return of ovarian function usually occurs following recovery from the infection.

More recently, there have been suggestions that human immune deficiency virus (HIV) infection (or anti retro viral therapy) can lead to POI [31]. There is a report of POI following human papilloma virus vaccination [32].

Environmental Toxins

Although there is no conclusive evidence, smoking may lead to POF. Female smokers experience menopause earlier than non-smokers suggesting a negative effect of smoking on ovarian function. An increased risk of POF has also been reported in women with epilepsy [33, 34].

Idiopathic

The idiopathic POF is a diagnosis of exclusion, and it is preferred when no other causes can be ascertained after complete evaluation. It is a label in about 75% to 90% of all women with POF [5].

Clinical Evaluation

Women with POF may present clinically in a variety of ways but the most common presentation is menstrual irregularities. They may present with a shortened or increased inter menstrual cycle interval. Menstrual irregularities include oligomenorrhea or amenorrhea, which is usually secondary amenorrhea, but a small percentage will present with primary amenorrhea and in these cases, a chromosomal cause is more likely. Usually, there are no symptoms and signs that precede the cessation of periods. They have normal menstrual history, age at menarche and possible fertility prior to the onset of POF.

Symptoms of estrogen deficiency may be noted such as hot flushes, vaginal dryness, and mood disturbances although delayed. Long-term consequences of hypo-estrogenism, which include osteoporosis, accelerated cardiovascular aging and neurocognitive disorders could also be experienced by these women [1].

Infertility is another consequence of POF that may be the clinical presentation. It is very distressing, as women with POF are faced with an unexpected and abrupt diagnosis following evaluation for oligo/amenorrhea even before they have attempted conception unlike most cases where couples discover they are infertile after several attempts at conception.

Some women may present with features of autoimmune disease and others with psychological symptoms as a consequence of the POF.

It is advisable to take a complete history and perform a thorough physical examination to exclude secondary causes of amenorrhea. These include pregnancy, polycystic ovary syndrome, hypothalamic amenorrhea, chronic medical illness secondary to poorly controlled diabetes or celiac disease, lifestyle habits (extreme exercise, poor caloric intake), hypothalamic or pituitary lesions, hyperprolactinaemia, hypo and hyperthyroidism. The screening history should also focus on a family history of POF, previous ovarian or pelvic surgery, viral infection, chemotherapy and radiotherapy, which may identify a cause [35]. The clinician should enquire about a personal or family history of autoimmune disorders - history of delayed puberty, delayed developmental milestones, mental retardation, intellectual disability, dry eyes and hearing impairment [5].

The physical examination should focus on body habitus especially to rule out Turner's syndrome. Evidence of normal secondary sexual characteristics, as well as evidence of vaginal atrophy secondary to hypo-estrogenism should be looked out for.

Investigation

There is a lack of standardized diagnostic criteria for POF, which results in diagnostic confusion. A study showed that over 50% of patients with POF had seen at least 3 clinicians before the diagnosis was made and in 25% the diagnosis took more than 5 years [36]. The following investigations are recommended but are by no means exhaustive. (Box 1)

Hormone Profile

It is the norm that estimation of gonadotrophin levels should be performed after 3-4 months of amenorrhea (secondary) or menstrual irregularity. In women younger than 40 years, at least two menopausal follicle stimulating hormone (FSH) levels (>40 IU/L) will be sufficient for the diagnosis of POF. Ideally it should be repeated after 4 weeks along with estradiol levels to confirm hypogonadism. Thyroid function tests and prolactin assays are also recommended to exclude alternative pathology. Basal luteinizing hormone (LH) measurement is assayed with the aim of evaluating the presence of functional follicles. Overall, if estradiol is above 50 pg/mL and LH level is above the level of FSH, it is an indication that there are at least several live follicles. Another diagnostic test gaining increasing interest is anti-Mullerian hormone (AMH). It is thought to be the most reliable measure of reduced ovarian reserve and may play a role in predicting age at menopause [37]. Unlike FSH, which is measured in the follicular phase of the menstrual cycle, AMH has the advantage that it can be measured at any time in the menstrual cycle.

Box 1. Investigations for POF

- *Hormone profile*: FSH, LH, AMH, Estradiol, Prolactin, Thyroid function tests
- *Autoimmune screen*: Anti-adrenal, anti-thyroid and anti-ovarian antibodies. For autoimmune thyroid disease additional anti-thyroid peroxidase and anti-thyroglobulin antibodies. *Ovarian biopsy
- *Karyotyping and genetic analysis*: 45 XO, FMR1 pre mutation, BMP15, FIGLA, GDF9, NR5A1 genes isolated
- *Pelvic ultrasonography*: AFC, ovarian volume and ovarian blood flow measurement using Doppler ultrasonography.
- *DXA scan*

*Ovarian biopsy is gold standard for diagnosing autoimmune POF but it is not recommended.

Autoimmune Screen

These tests will identify an underlying autoimmune cause or highlight those at increased risk of developing autoimmune disorders in the future. They include anti-adrenal, anti-thyroid and anti-ovarian antibodies. It is important to investigate the anti-adrenal antibodies, as patients with POF develop adrenal insufficiency 300 times more often than the general population [38]. Also, in terms of autoimmune thyroid diseases, it is appropriate to carry out thyroid function tests such as measurement of TSH, free T4, anti-thyroid-peroxidase and anti-thyroglobulin antibodies. Further tests may be carried out depending on other clinical suspicions such as galactosemia. The gold standard for determining autoimmune POF is ovarian biopsy, which is not recommended due to its unknown clinical value, expense and risks [9].

Karyotyping and Genetic Analysis

This is especially important in younger patients, those with primary amenorrhea or those with a family history of POF or learning difficulties to exclude an underlying genetic cause. The most common genetic disorders tested include X chromosome abnormalities, FMR1 pre mutation and the more recently identified BMP15, FIGLA, GDF9 and NR5A1 gene mutations [39]. More recently it has been suggested that patients with POF of unknown cause should be assessed in terms of FMR1 pre mutation [40].

Pelvic Ultrasonography

Ultrasonographic assessment of ovarian aging include antral follicle count (AFC), ovarian volume and ovarian blood flow measurement. The clinically most widely used is AFC. Doppler ultrasonography may show decreasing stromal blood flow in women with diminished ovarian reserve and can be used in future as a marker of premature aging. Ultrasound is also useful in diagnosing polycystic ovaries, which should be excluded as a cause of secondary amenorrhea. Ultrasound is important in the identification of the internal genitalia of those with primary amenorrhea and also, if necessary to display the streak gonads.

Dual-Energy X-Ray Absorptiometry (DXA) Scan

This is for estimation of baseline bone mineral density. Due to decreased estrogen levels, women with POF do not achieve peak bone density and may experience loss of bone mass. If hormone therapy is commenced and the woman has not experienced fractures, it is not necessary to do bone mineral density testing.

MANAGEMENT

The management of POF requires a multidisciplinary approach involving specialists such as consultant gynecologists, endocrinologists, psychologists, menopause nurse specialists, psychosexual counselors, dieticians and pharmacists to address their complex physical and psychological needs.

Initiation and management of hormone replacement therapy, contraception or fertility management, psychological support and annual screening to assess thyroid function, adrenal function and routine preventive health care are some components of proper management of these women.

Lifestyle Modification

General lifestyle modification and dietary measures are recommended to reduce the risk of developing osteoporosis and cardiovascular diseases which are some of the long term consequences of POF that may result in increased mortality among these women compared to their counterparts with a menopause after the age of 50 years. Regular exercises especially strength training exercise, cessation of smoking and reduction of intake of alcohol and caffeine will be useful. Referral to a dietician will help the women optimize their dietary intake. 1000mg of calcium and 800IU of vitamin D daily, as supplements are recommended. Supplementation is needed especially in those with reduced bone density.

Hormone Replacement Therapy (HRT)

Exogenous hormone replacement therapy (HRT) should be recommended to patients to prevent or provide relief from menopausal symptoms, bone mineral density loss, and deterioration in cardiovascular endothelial function. In adolescents, HRT is required to help induce secondary sexual characteristics. Options for hormone replacement include use of HRT or combined oral contraceptive pills (COCP). Women with POF need higher doses of estrogen than older postmenopausal women. It is more appropriate to give exogenous estrogen and cyclic progesterone to POF patients and it is advocated that HRT regime be continued until at least the average age of natural menopause (51 years) although there are no studies to support the optimal length of time they should be administered [35]. Currently, no evidence exists to support a particular route of administration or treatment regimen so cases should be individualized, taking into consideration the patient's choice.

Androgen replacement is given to women with POF especially those suffering from testosterone deficiency and exhibiting symptoms like lethargy or reduced libido. Serum testosterone levels should be kept within physiological limits to reduce risks of side effects such as acne and unwanted hair [41]. For those requiring HRT after malignancy or after treatment especially of hormone-sensitive tumors, it is best to liaise with the oncology team and consider delay in commencing HRT so as to help reduce the recurrence of the tumour.

Follow up visits for those on HRT are scheduled at 6 -12 month intervals with periodic testing of thyroid-stimulating hormone, calcium and cortisol levels. If anti-adrenal antibodies are present, an adrenocorticotropic stimulation test to assess adrenal reserve or referral to an endocrinologist is advised [35].

Contraception

The patients taking HRT should be warned that it is not a contraceptive if they do not wish to get pregnant. After diagnosis, spontaneous ovulation may occur in 25% of POF patients, and pregnancy may occur in 10%, regardless of the treatment [42]. Occurrence of ovulation and indeed conception in these women under such treatment with high doses of steroids is not yet understood. It is recommended that barrier methods be used despite HRT if the women do not want to become pregnant. The levonorgestrel intrauterine system (Mirena) may be used for both contraception and endometrial protection in association with estrogen as a continuous preparation. Evidence for this approach is minimal though [43].

Non-Hormonal Treatments

These are desirable when estrogen replacement is contraindicated as in patients with endometrial cancer or estrogen receptor-positive breast cancer or women at high risk of venous thromboembolism. It involves the use of complementary therapies, selective serotonin re-uptake inhibitors (SSRIs), gabapentin or venlafaxine. These provide symptomatic relief but will not reduce the long-term adverse consequences of hypo estrogenism. An informed decision is made before they can be used.

Fertility Preservation

Options for fertility preservation are offered to women undergoing chemotherapy or radiotherapy prior to initiation of treatment. These include ovarian hyperstimulation with oocyte retrieval followed by oocyte or embryo cryopreservation, ovarian tissue cryopreservation - still experimental although getting popular [44], or ovarian suppression with gonadotropin-releasing hormone agonist. Laparoscopic ovarian transposition before pelvic radiotherapy has also been used to prevent ovarian failure [42]. Unfortunately, the chances of success of ART in patients with POF are low. The fertility treatment with the highest success rate has been *in-vitro* fertilization with use of donor oocytes. This has been associated with a live birth rate of approximately 30% - 40% per embryo transferred [35]. It is noteworthy that these options are not all available in some centers and some techniques are still considered as experimental thus limiting the management of the infertility component.

Psychological and Psychosexual Support

Women with POF may experience significant psychological disturbance such as anxiety, depression and somatization with reduced self-esteem and overall life satisfaction [41]. They may also experience sexual dysfunction with reduced sexual wellbeing, reduced arousal and reduced frequency of sexual intercourse. Psychological support should be provided with regards to infertility, altered self-image and sexual dysfunction. They may require referral to psychologists and support groups.

Conclusion

Premature ovarian failure remains a poorly understood condition with complex physical adverse effects as well as long-term consequences of hypo-estrogenism, such as cardiovascular disease, neurocognitive decline, menopausal symptoms, osteoporosis and infertility. It is important to expedite the correct diagnosis and identify associated medical conditions so as to reduce these adverse consequences. A comprehensive multidisciplinary approach to management, which includes provision of hormone replacement therapy, physical or emotional support and fertility preservation, should be adopted. These women would also require preventive maintenance therapy and periodic surveillance as long-term follow-up.

References

[1] McKinlay, SM; Brambilla, DJ; Posner, JG. The normal menopause transition. *Maturitas.*, 1992, 14, 103-115.

[2] Miro, F; Parker, SW; Aspinall, LJ; Coley, J; Perry, PW; Ellis, JE. Sequential classification of endocrine stages during reproductive aging in women: the FREEDOM study. *Menopause.*, 2005, 12, 281-290.

[3] Kalu, E; Panay, N. Spontaneous premature ovarian failure: management challenges. *Gynecol Endocrinol.*, 2008, 24, 273-279.

[4] Albright, F; Smith, PH; Fraser, R. A syndrome characterized by primary ovarian insufficiency and decreased stature. *Am J Med Sci.*, 1942, 204, 625-648.

[5] Nelson, LM. Clinical practice. Primary ovarian insufficiency. *N Engl J Med.*, 2009, 360, 606-614.

[6] Welt, CK. Primary ovarian insufficiency: a more accurate term for premature ovarian failure. *Clin Endocrinol.*, 2008, 68, 499-509.

[7] Coulam, CB; Adamson, SC; Annegers, JF. Incidence of premature ovarian failure. *Obstet Gynecol*, 1986, 67, 604-606.

[8] Rafique, S; Sterling, E; Lawrence, N. A new approach to primary ovarian insufficiency. *Obstet Gynecol Clin N Am.*, 2012, 39, 567-586.

[9] Goswani, D; Conway, GS. Premature ovarian failure. *Hum Reprod Update.*, 2005, 11(4), 391-410.

[10] Hook, EB; Warbuton, D. The distribution of chromosomal genotypes associated with Turner's syndrome: livebirth prevalence rates and evidence for diminished fetal mortality and severity in genotypes associated with structural X abnormalities or mosaicism. *Hum Genet.*, 1983, 64(1), 24-27.

[11] Holland, CM. 47, XXX in an adolescent with premature ovarian failure and autoimmune disease. *J Pediatr Adolesc Gynecol.*, 2001, 14(2), 77-80.

[12] Goswami, R; Goswami, D; Kabara, M; Gupta, N; Dubey, S; Dadhwal, V. Prevalence of the triple X syndrome in phenotypically normal women with premature ovarian failure and its association with autoimmune thyroid disorders. *Fertil Steril.*, 2003, 80 (4), 1052-1054.

[13] Rooman, RP; Van Driessche, K; Du Caju, MV. Growth and ovarian function in girls with 48, XXXX karyotype – patient report and review of literature. *J Pediatr Endocrinol Metab.*, 2002, 15(7), 1051-1055.

[14] Mahbod, E; Firoozeh, AA. Pathogenesis and Causes of Premature Ovarian Failure: An Update. *Int J Fertil Steril.*, 2011, 5(2), 54-65.

[15] Biancalana, V; Beldjord, C; Taillandier, A; Szpiro-Tapia, S; Cusin, V; Gerson, F; et al. Five years of molecular diagnosis of fragile X syndrome (1997-2001): a collaborative study reporting 95% of the activity in France. *Am J Med Genet.*, 2004, 129A(3), 218-224.

[16] Persani, L; Rossetti, R; Cacciatore, C; Bonomi, M. Primary ovarian insufficiency: X chromosome defects and autoimmunity. *J Autoimmun.*, 2009, 33, 35-41.

[17] Shelling, AN. Premature ovarian failure. *Reprod.*, 2010, 140, 633-641.

[18] Bakalov, VK; Anasti, JN; Calis, KA; Vanderhoof, VH; Premkumar, A; Chen, S; et al. Autoimmune oophoritis as a mechanism of follicular dysfunction in women with 46, XX spontaneous premature ovarian failure. *Fertil Steril.*, 2005, 84(4), 958-965.

[19] Lebovic, DI; Naz, R. Premature ovarian failure: Think aȍutoimmune disorder. *Sexual Reprod Menop.*, 2004, 2(4), 230-233.

[20] Falorni, A; Laureti, S; Candeloro, P; Perrino, S; Coronella, C; Bizzarro, A; et al. Steroid -cell autoantibodies are preferentially expressed in women with premature ovarian failure who have adrenal autoimmunity. *Fertil Steril.*, 2002, 78(2), 270-279.

[21] La Barbera, AR; Miller, MM; Ober, C; Rebar, RW. Autoimmune aetiology in premature ovarian failure. *Am J Reprod Immunol Microbiol.*, 1988, 16, 115-122.

[22] Hoeck, A; Schoemaker, J; Dreshage, HA. Premature ovarian failure and ovarian autoimmunity. *Endocr Rev.*, 1997, 18, 107-134.

[23] Blumenfeld, Z; Eckman, A. Preservation of fertility and ovarian function and minimization of gonadotoxicity in young women by GnRH-a. *J Natl Cancer Inst Monogr.*, 2005, 34, 40-43.
[24] Beerendonk, CC; Braat DD. Present and future options for the preservation of fertility in female adolescents with cancer. *Endocr Dev.*, 2005, 8, 166-175.
[25] Morice, P; Thiam-Ba, R; Castaigne, D; Haie-Meder, C; Gerbaulet, A; Pautier, P; et al. Fertility results after ovarian transposition for pelvic malignancies treated by external irradiation or brachytherapy. *Hum Reprod.*, 1998, 13, 660-663.
[26] Longway, M; Matthews, CA. Resumption of ovarian function 20 years after chemotherapy-induced ovarian failure: A case report. *Fertil Steril.*, 2009, 92(1), 392 e17-e18.
[27] Wikstorm, AM; Hovi, L; Dunkel, L; Saarinen-Pihkala, UM. Restoration of ovarian function after chemotherapy for osteosarcoma. *Arch Dis Child.*, 2003, 88(5), 428-431.
[28] Green, DM; Sklar, CA; Boice, JD; Jr. Mulvihill, JJ; Whitton, JA; Stovall, M; et al. Ovarian failure and reproductive outcomes after childhood cancer treatment: results from the childhood cancer survivor study. *J Clin Oncol.*, 2009, 27(14), 2374-2381.
[29] Panay, N; Kalu, E. Management of premature ovarian failure. *Best Prac Res Clin Obstet Gynecol.*, 2009, 23(1), 129-140.
[30] Rees, M; Purdie, D. Premature menopause: Management of the menopause: the handbook. 4th ed. London: Royal Society of Medicine Press Ltd. 2006, 142-149.
[31] Ohi, J; Partisani, M; Demangeat, C; Binder-Foucard, F; Nisand, I; Lang, JM. Alterations of ovarian reserve tests in human immunodeficiency virus (HIV) – infected women. *Gynecol Obstet Fertil.*, 2010, 38, 313-317.
[32] Little, DT; Ward, HRG. Adolescent premature ovarian insufficiency following Human pappiloma virus vaccination. A case series seen in general practice. *Journal of Investigative medicine HIGH IMPACT CASE REPORTS.*, 2014, 2(4), 2324709614556129.
[33] Chang, SH; Kim, CS; Lee, KS; Kim, H; Yim, SV; Lim, YJ; Park, SK. Premenopausal factors influencing premature ovarian failure and early menopause. *Maturitas.*, 2007, 58(1), 19-30.
[34] Klevin, P; Serje, A; Pezzullo, JC. Premature ovarian failure in women with epilepsy. *Epilepsia.*, 2001, 42(12), 1584-1589.
[35] Cox, L; Liu, JH. Primary ovarian insufficiency: an update. *Int J Womens Health.*, 2014, 6, 235-243.
[36] Alzubaidi, NH; Chapin, HL; Vanderhoof, VH; Callis, CA; Nelson, LM. Meeting the needs of young women with secondary amenorrhea and spontaneous premature ovarian failure. *Obstet Gynaecol.*, 2002, 99, 720-725.
[37] Tehrani, A; Shakeri, N; Azizi, F. Whether age at menopause is predictable using serum anti-Mullerian hormone concentration? *Hum Reprod.*, 2010, 25, i1-i3.
[38] Bakalov, VK; Vanderhoof, VH; Bondy, CA; Nelson, LM. Adrenal antibodies detect asymptomatic autoimmune adrenal insufficiency in young women with spontaneous premature ovarian failure. *Hum Reprod.*, 2002, 17, 2096-2100.
[39] Persani, L; Rossetti, R; Cacciatore, C. Genes involved in human premature ovarian failure. *J Mol Endocrinol.*, 2010, 45, 257-279.

[40] American College of Obstetricians and Gynecologists Committee on Genetics. ACOG committee opinion. No. 338: Screening for fragile X syndrome. *Obstet Gynecol.*, 2006, 107, 1483-1485.

[41] van der Stege, JG; Groen, H; van Zaldelhoff, SJ; et al. Decreased androgen concentrations and diminished general and sexual well-being in women with premature ovarian failure. *Menopause.*, 2008, 15, 23-31.

[42] Sukur, YE; Kivancli, IB; Ozmen, B. Ovarian aging and premature ovarian failure. *J Turk Ger Gynecol Assoc.*, 2014, 15(3), 190-196.

[43] Maclaran, K; Panay, N. Premature ovarian failure *J Fam Plann Reprod Health Care.*, 2010, 37, 35-42.

[44] Şükür, YE; Özmen, B; Sönmezer, M. Cancer and ovarian tissue cryopreservation. *Turk J Med Sci.*, 2010, 40, 159–168.

[45] Cooper, AR; Baker, VL; Sterling, EW; Ryan, ME; Woodruff, TK; Nelson, LM. The time is now for a new approach to primary ovarian insufficiency. *Fertil Steril.*, 2011, 95(6), 1890-1897.

In: Amenorrhea
Editor: Oliver Chukwujekwu Ezechi
ISBN: 978-1-63484-778-0

Chapter 15

FEMALE ATHLETE TRIAD

Oliver Chukwujekwu Ezechi
Division of Clinical Sciences, Nigerian Institute of Medical Research,
Yaba Lagos, Nigeria

ABSTRACT

The female athlete triad (FAT) is a spectrum of interrelated pathophysiologic consequences of low energy availability, menstrual dysfunction, and low bone mineral density as a result of excessive physical activity. The components of the triad are not only counterproductive to goals of athletic performance, but often lead to serious long term negative health outcomes. Presence of one component of the spectrum requires screening for the remaining two. The prevention of the potentially severe consequences of FAT requires early detection of the disorder and vigilance of health workers that work with athletes.

Keywords: female athlete triad disordered eating, menstrual dysfunction, altered bone density, low energy

INTRODUCTION

Good health and general wellbeing is promoted by physical activity and thus recommended for all ages. However, despite the numerous health benefits of physical activity and exercise, there are also negative consequences of excessive physical activity especially in women and girls. Female athletes are particularly at risk for these negative outcomes, prompting the American College of sports medicine in 1992 to coin the term Female Athlete Triad [1, 2]. The original definition of FAT as a syndromes consisting of amenorrhea, disordered eating and osteoporosis was updated in 1997 to include a spectrum of dysfunction related to menstrual function, energy availability and bone mineral density. An athlete condition can therefore fall anywhere along the spectrum of optimal energy availability to an eating disorder, menstrual regularity to subclinical menstrual disorders, orthorexia, or amenorrhea; and low bone mineral density to frank osteoporosis [1].

The International Olympic Committee, in keeping with its role to protect athletes, in 2005 convened an expert committee to evaluate the entity known as FAT. The Consensus statement defined FAT as 'the combination of disordered eating and irregular menstrual cycles eventually leading to a decrease in endogenous oestrogen and other hormones, resulting in low bone mineral density'[3]. The American College of Sports Medicine in 2007, following progress in scientific understanding of the entity, redefined FAT as a clinical entity that refers to the 'relationship between three interrelated components: energy availability (EA), menstrual function and bone health.' It further recognised that over a period of time, an athlete can move along the continuous spectrum ranging from the healthy athlete with optimal EA, regular menses and healthy bones to the opposite end of the spectrum characterised by amenorrhea, low EA and osteoporosis [2]. Emerging scientific evidence and clinical experience show that the aetiological factor underpinning FAT is an energy deficiency relative to the balance between dietary energy intake (EI) and the energy expenditure required to support homoeostasis, health and the activities of daily living, growth and sporting activities. It is increasingly becoming evident that the clinical entity called FAT is not a triad of three entities after all, rather a syndrome resulting from relative energy deficiency that affects many aspects of physiological function including metabolic rate, menstrual function, bone health, immunity, protein synthesis, cardiovascular and psychological health [1-3]. In addition, the reported relative energy deficiency in female athletes, also affects men, making the terminology FAT a misnomer. A new terminology that will encompass all the entities as well as take into account that it also occur in males was therefore needed. The IOC interdisciplinary experts introduce a more comprehensive and broader term for the syndrome called "Relative Energy Deficiency in Sport (RED-S)." RED-S refers to impaired physiological function including, but not limited to, metabolic rate, menstrual function, bone health, immunity, protein synthesis and cardiovascular health caused by relative energy deficiency [3].

EPIDEMIOLOGY

A wide variation in the prevalence of all three component of the triad ranging from 0 – 15.9% has been report [4]. This wide variation has been attributed to several factors, including the changing definition of FAT, type of sport, age of athlete, as well as inherent diagnostic challenges. It is unusual for all components of the triad to be diagnosed in tandem, as athlete afflicted with the triad evolve symptoms and features of FAT along non-consistent continuums for each component of the triad. Female athlete participating in sports that assign age classification and aesthetic value to performance like gymnastics, Judo, wrestling, ballet dancing, and ice skating are at higher risk for developing the syndrome [4].

The lack or poor collection of routine data from athlete especially in low and middle income countries makes it difficult to have correct and exact national, regional and global epidemiologic data on FAT. The practice of athlete to hide their symptoms, habits or behaviour from significant persons is also another contributor to the drought of information on FAT. This reluctance accounts for the reported difficulty in diagnosing the condition and late presentation of athlete only in advanced stage of the illness, when the symptoms are obvious. Lack of awareness and poor knowledge about FAT on the part of physicians makes it difficult to diagnosis mild cases.

The estimated prevalence of FAT is generally low, but the individual components of the triad are common in athletes at all ages and levels of competition [5]. A meta-analysis conducted by Gibbs JC et al. in 2013 reported a low prevalence range of 0-15.9% of FAT among athlete across all levels of sporting activities [4]. In the study, the prevalence of individual components of triad was noted to be higher, ranging from 2.7% to 27.9% and 16.0% to 60.0% respectively for any 2 or any 1 of the triad components respectively [4]. Nattiv A et al. reporting in the American College of Sports Medicine position noted that occurs FAT 2 to 3 higher in sports that emphasise weight category or aesthetics than in non-lean sports [6]. Disordered eating among female athlete has been estimated to be as high as 62%, with the incidence of bulimia and anorexia nervosa estimated at 4-39%. The menstrual dysfunction component of the triad is difficult to assess, however, a prevalence ranging from 6% to 79% has been reported in various studies and varied according to the definition and assessment adopted for menstrual dysfunction, type of sport, age of athlete, use of contraceptives, volume of training, and the presence of subclinical menstrual disorders [1, 3, 5, 6]. Altered bone mineral density (BMD) have been found to be increased in most athletes compared to sedentary controls, but low BMD often is seen in amenorrheic athletes. Khan KM et al. reported that 22% to 50% of amenorrheic athletes had osteopenia compared to 12% in controls [7]. Osteoporosis was also found to be higher among these group of athletes (13%) compared to controls (2.3%) [9]. Despite lack of epidemiologic clarity, the association between these three disorders is well established, meriting evaluation of all components of the triad when one disorder is identified [1-6].

PATHOGENESIS

Insufficient energy to supply metabolic demand is the primary disorder driving pathophysiologic changes in FAT. Deficient energy balance results in insufficient metabolic supply for normal menstrual function, bone development, and bone maintenance. Caloric intake, baseline metabolic function, and energy expenditure are factors that dictate available energy [1-5].

Low Energy

Energy restriction is common in sport, and for many athletes it is necessary to achieve the sport-specific bodyweight and composition that result in optimum performance. Female athletes' drive to ensure that the specific bodyweight is achieved and the importance of fat loss, consume 30% less energy per unit of bodyweight than male athletes [1, 3, 5]. This often leads female athletes to engage in disordered eating, involving dietary restriction and purgative behaviours such as vomiting and misuse of laxatives. This is most common in sports in which low bodyweight conveys a competitive advantage. Energy availability is the dietary energy left in the body after completion of exercise. Low energy availability is not synonymous with disordered eating; rather it may be the result from either reduced caloric intake or increased energy output. Athlete who increase their training requirements, also need to increase their caloric intake in other to avoid energy deficiency. It is the decreased caloric intake component that may be common between disordered eating and low energy availability [1, 2].

Low energy irrespective of the causative mechanism leads to hormonal abnormalities that may exacerbate other triad symptoms. Restriction of energy results in the body conserving energy by altering body metabolism. The alteration in body metabolism is achieved through the suppression of gonadotropin-releasing hormone pulsatility and disruption of the number of pulses of luteinizing hormone (LH) and follicle-stimulating hormone (FSH). This further leads to a decrease in oestrogen levels [8]. The decreased body fat as a result of restriction of dietary fat and increased training results in decrease in leptin which play a role in the normal menstrual cycle. Short-term ghrelin dysregulation as a result of disordered eating can self-perpetuate and a vicious cycle result with long-term consequences. The intestinally derived anorexigen peptide YY is elevated [9]. in severe weight loss as a result of disordered eating which has been shown to contribute to bone loss. Disordered eating also lead to of androgen deficiency and elevation of cortisol, both of which are factors in energy metabolism and maintenance of bone density [10].

Menstrual Dysfunction

Menstrual dysfunction may present as primary amenorrhea, secondary amenorrhea, or oligomenorrhea. The causes of menstrual dysfunction are not well-defined, but most likely multi factorial. Exercise and its energy demands, if not compensated by adequate nutrition, may affect several cerebral neuro-transmitters and, subsequently, the hormones of the hypothalamic-pituitary-ovarian axis. These hormonal changes may be reflected as luteal phase deficiency, anovulatory cycles, or amenorrhea [1].

Excessive exercise in the face of inadequate caloric and nutritional replacement leads to a negative energy balance that affects cerebral neuro-transmitters and the hypothalamic-pituitary-ovarian hormonal system. Energy balance is very important for menstrual function, and it has been suggested that the dysfunction in menstruation is an adaptive response to the negative energy balance [3, 10, 11]. The resulting low energy causes the body to stop reproductive function to preserve energy for more vital functions [3, 10]. The gonadotropin-releasing hormone (GnRH) pulse generator is suppressed. Excessive exercise alters many hormones that affect the GnRH pulse generator. These include the catecholamines, cortisol, dopamine, endorphins, prostaglandins, catecholestrogens and serotonin. These hormones in turn affect the release of follicle stimulating (FSH) and Luteinizing hormones (LH), and thus estrogen and progesterone. The long-term consequences of this reversible suppression of the GnRH pulse generator include infertility, bone density loss, stress fractures, and increased injuries [1].

Altered Bone Mineral Density

The third component of FAT, altered bone mineral density ranges from optimal bones health to osteoporosis [1]. It focuses on bone strength, which consists of bone mineral density and bone quality. A continuous process of balanced osteoblastic and osteclastic activity is required for the maintance of bone health. In a healthy menstruating female, the normal oestrogen levels suppress osteclastic activity resulting in bone development and normal bone mineral density. In FAT, the negative energy balance alters the GnRH pulsatility, which further suppresses the hypothalamic-pituitary axis. The resulting hypoestrogenic state suppresses osteoblast formations and increase in osteclastic activity which alters bone mineral density. The development and maintenance of bone health in preferential anatomic locations are altered by rigorous athletic activity. Sport activity in female athletes may increase density of weight bearing bones, while the non-weight bearing bones like spine may show altered bone mineral density [6, 12, 13]. The bones of pelvis, vertebrae and the lower limbs, are most commonly affected by poor bone health in women with the FAT. Female athlete involved in high impact sports are more susceptible to fractures than their nonathletic and menstruating athletic counterparts while they lose 1.5% of bone mineral density per year the others gain about 3% of bone mass per year [6, 13].

Other Dysfunction in FAT

Many psychological and physiological dysfunctions that affect other body systems have been found in female athletes with FAT [3]. This includes chronic fatigue, increased risk of infection and illness, electrolyte imbalance, decrease production of growth hormone, unfavourable lipid profiles, endothelial dysfunction, and depression. Emerging evidence do suggest that the FAT is not a triad but a tetrad of interconnected conditions [3]. Endothelial dysfunction is the new emerging component, resulting from a decrease in estrogen following chronic low energy availability [3]. The suggested new component is concerning because the sentinel event in pathogenesis of cardiovascular disease is impaired endothelial function.

Risk Factors

Several dietary, exercise related and psychosocial behaviours are associated with increased risk of FAT [1]. Restriction of dietary energy intake, limitation of type of food intake and vegetarian diet are some of the dietary behaviour that has been found to predispose female athlete to FAT. Exercise for prolonged period of time, initiation of training at young age or increase in intensity of training, participation in lean and aesthetic sports are some of the exercise related behaviour that may be associated with FAT. Psychosocial pressures to achieve thinness, low self-esteem or poor family dynamics also may predispose athlete to development of FAT.

Athletes with low body mass index or participate in lean/aesthetic sports are at risk for at risk for menstrual dysfunction. However, exercise alone has no suppressive effect on pulsatility of luteinizing hormone (LH) when energy intake is increased to compensate for energy expenditure [1, 14]. Low bone mineral density, menstrual dysfunction, late onset of menstruation, dietary insufficiency, genetic predisposition and bone structure type are some of the risk factors for stress fracture [14-17]. The observation of mood changes, dissatisfaction with body size, and decline in performance, frequent illness, injury or fractures [1, 14-17] are warning signs for the development of FAT.

EVALUATION

A detailed screening history should be obtained from an athlete identified as being at risk for FAT. The screening process entails obtaining information on the patient's medical, dietary and exercise history. She should also be evaluated for existing psychopathology and medical complications. A multidisciplinary approach is recommended in the evaluation of patient with FAT. Consultation should be extended to the psychiatrist or clinical psychologist, an orthopedic surgeon, a cardiologist, nutritionist and the athlete's physical trainer [1, 12].

A detailed and thorough medical history, include endocrine deficiencies past, stress fractures and complete fractures. Menstrual history should include age of onset, length of menstrual flow and cycle, pattern of menstruation and missed periods especially during the peak of sporting activities. Explore the possible use of steroid as the cause of the amenorrhea, as some athletes may use them to enhance their strength. Always do exclude pregnancy, as it is the most common cause of secondary amenorrhea in women of reproductive age group. Athlete's psychosocial history is important as it may be a pointer to her challenge. The lack of family or social support system is a risk factor for FAT. The patients exercise routine need to be reviewed in details. The physician should routinely ask how much time is spent in formal practice and how much additional time apart from scheduled workouts is spent on other related activities during off-season or if it continues year round. Detailed nutritional history should be take and their calorie contents obtained and compared with amount spent on exercise. History should include the use of any prescription medications, including contraceptive and any herbal remedies or nutritional supplements [1, 12].

Many validated tools exist for the evaluation of the component of triad and should be used during evaluation. This include the Athletic Milieu Direct Questionnaire, the Female Athlete Screening Tool, the American Physiological Screening Test for eating disorders among Female College Athletes and the Low Energy Availability in Females Questionnaire [1, 12].

COMPLICATIONS

Irreversible osteoporosis is the most worrisome complication of the FAT, as a result of continuous bone mineral density loss. Osteoarthritis could result from multiple stress fractures or complete fractures. Fractures in women with FAT tend take longer to heal as a result of the negative nutritional balance. Other complications include anorexia, prolonged hospitalization, cardiac arrhythmias, or even death. Psychological and physiological dysfunctions affecting virtually all the systems have been reported. Anaemia, chronic fatigue, esophagitis, electrolyte imbalance, slowing of the metabolic rate, decreased production of growth hormone, unfavorable lipid panels, endothelial dysfunction, reduced muscle protein synthesis, increased risk of infection and ill health, and depression are other complications of FAT [7, 11, 13].

Laboratory Investigation

Diagnosis of FAT is largely clinical; no test confirms the diagnosis. Laboratory investigations should include pregnancy test, dual-energy x-ray absorptiometry, magnetic resonance imaging, pelvic ultrasound, bone scanning, electrocardiography, progesterone challenge, or endometrial biopsy. Other tests include liver function, electrolyte levels, and kidney function, thyroid function test to exclude hyperthyroidism and hypothyroidism. FSH and LH to evaluate pituitary function and possible premature ovarian failure [1, 12, 7].

Treatment

The adoption of a multidisciplinary approach in the management of FAT is the key to a successful treatment of an athlete with the condition. At a minimum the team should include a physician, a dietitian, a mental health professional and a gynaecologist. In a well-resourced setting additional supportive role should be taken by physical therapists, coaches, and family members. The athlete should be made to know that food is as important and the energy needed for her performance [1, 12].

Prevention

Athletes, coaches and primary physicians should be educated on the symptoms, risk factors and complications of FAT. This will assist in early identification of persons at risk, the condition and initiation of treatment on time to prevent complications. The all-time saying that prevention is better and cheaper than cure is exemplified by the consequence of FAT when is allowed to occur in athletes.

Psychological Therapy

Athletes with severe eating disorder and those unable to adhere to the nutritional and exercise programme require the services of psychiatrist or clinical psychologist. Cognitive behavioural and family therapy have been shown to be beneficial.

Nutritional Therapy

Increasing energy availability through adequate diet that provides sufficient calories result in restoration of menstrual function and improvement in bone mineral density. In practical terms, athlete should aim to gain 1 to 2 kg or a 10% reduction in exercise. This is sufficient to restore menstruation and increases bone mineral density up to 5% per year. Early involvement of a dietitian is essential for a successful nutrition programme foe an athlete with FAT. The recommended energy intake for sedentary and active women is 1800 to 2000 kcal/day, and 2300 to 3000 kcal/day respectively. The athlete, coach and dietitian should develop a meal plan based on the sport, the type of exercise and built of the athlete. This plan should be followed rigidly.

Exercise Modification

Adjust in the exercise regimen to include weight training exercises have been reported to have positive effects on skeletal health. Often there is need to adjust down the total time spent on the training to allow for energy balance.

Drug Therapy

Rarely drug therapy can be used in athlete with FAT, especially those with eating disorders and obsessed with super performance and always wining mentality. Antidepressants and anxiolytics is the drug of choice for the mental health professional in managing this kind of patient. Optimization of calcium and vitamin D intake to 1300 mg/d and 800 to 1000 IU/respectively is recommended for athlete with skeletal health challenges. Ethinyl estradiol 20 to 30mg may be prescribed for athletes older than 16 years who have persistent primary or secondary amenorrhea if there evidence of decline in BMD despite adequate nutritional intake [1, 12, 13].

Conclusion

FAT is a spectrum of interrelated conditions often observed in athlete. It involves three components of low energy availability with or without disordered eating, menstrual dysfunction and low bone mineral density. Early intervention prevents progression to clinical eating disorders, amenorrhea and osteoporosis. It is essential that athletes at risk of the condition are detected early in the course of the condition. Detecting the disorder early is the most important factor for preventing the potentially severe consequences, and requires heightened vigilance on the part of all those who work with this special patient population.

REFERENCES

[1] Javed A., Tebben P. J., Fischer P. R., Lteif A. N. 2013, September). Female athlete triad and its components: toward improved screening and management. *In Mayo Clinic Proceedings* 2013; 88 (9): 996-1009).

[2] Otis C. L., Drinkwater B., Johnson M., Loucks A., Wilmore J. American College of Sports Medicine position stand: the Female Athlete Triad. *Med. Sci. Sports Exerc.* 1997; 29(5): i-ix.

[3] Mountjoy M, Sundgot-Borgen J, Burke L, et al. The IOC consensus statement: beyond the Female Athlete Triad--Relative Energy Deficiency in Sport (RED-S). *Br. J. Sports Med.* 2014;48(7): 491-502.

[4] Gibbs J. C., Williams N. I., De Souza MJ. Prevalence of individual and combined components of the female athlete triad. *Med. Sci. Sports* Exerc. 2013; 45(5): 985-996.

[5] Nichols D. L., Sanborn C F., Essery E. V. Bone density and young athletic women: an update. *Sports Med.* 2007; 37(11): 1001-1014.

[6] Nattiv A., Loucks A B., Manore MM, et al; American College of Sports Medicine. American College of Sports Medicine position stand: the female athlete triad. *Med. Sci. Sports Exerc.* 2007; 39(10): 1867-1882.

[7] Khan K. M., Liu-Ambrose T., Sran M. M., et al. New criteria for the female athlete triad syndrome? As osteoporosis is rare, should osteopenia be among the criteria for defining the female athlete triad syndrome? *Br. J. Sports Med.* 2002; 36: 10-13.

[8] Mendelsohn F.A., Warren M. P. Anorexia, bulimia, and the female athlete triad: evaluation and management. *Endocrinol. Metab. Clin. N. Am.* 2010; 39: 155-167.

[9] Misra M, Miller KK, Tsai P, et al. Elevated peptide YY levels in adolescent girls with anorexia nervosa. *J. Clin. Endocrinol. MeTable* 2006; 91: 1027-1033.

[10] Lawson EA, Klibanski A. Endocrine abnormalities in anorexia nervosa. *Nat. Clin. Pract. Endocrinol. MeTable* 2008; 4:407-414.

[11] Waldrop J. Early identification and interventions for female athlete triad. *J. Pediatr. Health Care*. Jul-Aug 2005; 19(4): 213-20.

[12] Horn E, Gergen N, McGarry KA. The Female Athlete Triad. *Rhode Island medical journal* 2014; 11: 18-21.

[13] De Souza M. J., Williams N.I. Beyond hypoestrogenism in amenorrheic athletes: energy deficiency as a contributing factor for bone loss. *Curr. Sports Med. Rep*. 2005; 4(1):38-44.

[14] BARROW G. W., and S. SAHA Menstrual irregularity and stress fractures in collegiate female distance runners. *Am. J. Sports Med.* 1988; 16:209–216.

[15] MYBURGH, K. H., J. HUTCHINS, A. B. FATAAR, S. F. HOUGH, and T. D. N OAKES. Low bone density is an etiologic factor for stress fractures in athletes. *Ann. Intern. Med.* 1990; 113: 754–759.

[16] Loucks, A. B., M. Verdun, and E. M. HEATH. Low energyavailability, not stress of exercise, alters LH pulsatility in exercising women. *J. Appl. Physiol.* 1998; 84:37–46.

[17] Sundgot -Borgen, J. Risk and trigger factors for the development of eating disorders in female elite athletes. *Med. Sci. Sports Exerc.* 1994; 26: 414–419.

In: Amenorrhea
Editor: Oliver Chukwujekwu Ezechi

ISBN: 978-1-63484-778-0

Chapter 16

MENSTRUAL ABNORMALITIES IN ANOREXIA NERVOSA

Megan E. Harrison, Amy Robinson and Mark L. Norris
University of Ottawa. Division of Adolescent Medicine,
Children's Hospital of Eastern Ontario, Ottawa, Canada

ABSTRACT

Menstrual dysfunction is a common feature of all eating disorder subtypes. In anorexia nervosa, patients often present with amenorrhea or oligomenorrhea. The menstrual abnormalities experienced by patients with anorexia nervosa are in general thought to be secondary to dysfunction of the hypothalamic-pituitary-ovarian axis, specifically hypothalamic hypogonadism. Although the exact mechanisms that lead to menstrual dysfunction are not clear, it is thought that the concentration and function of several hormones are affected by a variety of circumstances, including weight loss and/or weight fluctuations, decreased body fat percentage, severe weight control behaviours and psychological stressors. In addition to the impaired hypothalamic secretion of gonadotropin-releasing hormone and low levels of luteinizing hormone, follicular stimulating hormone and estradiol, low levels of the hormones leptin and insulin-like growth factor-1 have also been implicated in contributing to the menstrual abnormalities in patients with anorexia nervosa. The menstrual dysfunction and hormonal alterations seen in patients with anorexia nervosa can result in significant medical complications, such as growth restriction, pubertal delay, and insufficient bone mineral density accrual. As such, it is imperative that research exploring the mechanisms of menstrual dysfunction in eating disorders and its treatment continues to build in order to improve the outcomes in this population.

Keywords: anorexia nervosa, weight loss, menstrual irregularity, amenorrhea

INTRODUCTION

Anorexia nervosa (AN) is the third most common chronic illness affecting young females with an estimated prevalence rate of 0.3-0.6% [1-3]. With recent changes to the diagnostic criteria for AN [4], and with the knowledge that many patients do not seek treatment for their illness, this prevalence rate is likely an underestimate [1, 2]. AN is a serious psychiatric condition associated with significant morbidity and mortality [5-7]. Patients with AN commonly experience some degree of menstrual dysfunction as evidenced by DSM-IV's prior inclusion of amenorrhea as a necessary component for diagnosis, although research has more recently shown that there are few to no differences in overall clinical presentation (for example demographics, eating behaviours, and psychopathology) [8-12] or treatment outcomes [10, 12] in patients with AN who met the amenorrhea criteria and those with AN who did not. As such, the diagnostic criteria for AN was updated in DSM-5, and the requirement for amenorrhea to be present was removed [4]. Of note and importance, menstrual dysfunction and hormonal alterations seen in AN can adversely affect an individual's growth, pubertal progression, and bone mineral density accrual, which highlights the importance of early recognition and effective treatments.

CLINICAL PRESENTATION

The age of onset of AN is most commonly in mid to late adolescence, although age of onset has been decreasing over the past years [13, 14]. AN is known to be more common in females with a female to male ratio of 10:1 [2] although this ratio is likely an underestimate as eating disorders in males are largely under detected [15, 16]. Patients with AN have significant low body weight (in the context of what is minimally expected for age, sex, developmental trajectory, and physical health) secondary to energy restriction, a strong fear of weight gain or behaviours that interfere with weight gain, and disturbances in the way they experience their body weight/shape [4]. The condition affects all organ systems [5, 17] and carries with it an annual mortality of 5.10 deaths (95% CI, 3.99-6.14) per 1000 person-years, and a standardized mortality ratio of 5.86 (95% CI, 4.17-8.26) [7, 18] to 6.2 (95% CI 5.5–7.0) [19], the highest mortality rate of all psychiatric conditions.

Menstrual irregularities are a common presenting concern in patients with AN [20]. Individuals with eating disorders (including those with variants of AN as well as those with bulimia nervosa) can present with amenorrhea, oligomenorrhea or have normal menstrual function [21]. Due to the variability in menstrual presentation in those with eating disorders, menstrual status is not a reliable criteria to distinguish different types of EDs [21]. Common patterns of menstrual dysfunction in patients with AN include primary and secondary amenorrhea, as well as oligomenorrhea. In many cases, menstrual abnormalities occur prior to the onset of weight loss [22].

Patients with AN may have various findings on physical examination depending on the degree of weight loss, starvation, and compensatory behaviours such as self-induced vomiting. Signs of starvation and weight loss can include bradycardia, hypothermia, lanugo hair growth, a scaphoid abdomen secondary to a loss of subcutaneous fat and an overall emaciated appearance. On external female genital examination, patients with AN can, depending on the degree of malnutrition, have findings in keeping with hypoestrogenemia, such as a pre-pubertal vaginal mucosa [20]. Depending on their developmental status and age, individuals with AN may also present with growth stunting and delayed or halted puberty status. Physical exam findings consistent with ongoing or chronic purging may include swelling in the parotid glands and/or submandibular region, calluses on the knuckles of the hand that is used to self-induce purging (Russell's sign), and oral changes such as poor dentition and halitosis [23].

PATHOGENESIS

The menstrual dysfunction seen in AN is thought to be secondary to a disruption of the hypothalamic-pituitary-ovarian (HPO) axis that results in a decrease in gonadotropin-releasing hormone (GnRH) secretion and subsequently low levels of luteinizing hormone (LH) and follicular-stimulating hormone (FSH), otherwise known as hypothalamic hypogonadism [20, 24-26]. The low levels of circulating gonadotropins (LH, FSH) lead to a decrease in estrogen levels in the context of a dysfunctional hypothalamic response to the normal positive feedback mechanisms of estrogen [27]. As a result, malnourished individuals with AN often exhibit a prepubertal pulsatile secretion pattern of LH [26], and overall suppressed levels of gonadotropins and estradiol [24].

The etiology of the hypothalamic dysfunction that leads to amenorrhea and menstrual dysfunction in AN is not completely understood, however multiple variables have been implicated in its pathogenesis and will be discussed below. Almost certainly the pathogenesis is multifactorial and involves a combination factors.

The Role of Body Weight

Absolute weight is thought to be essential in maintaining a normal menstrual cycle. Correspondingly, women with eating disorders and amenorrhea have been found to have a significantly lower weight than those with eating disorders without amenorrhea [9, 12, 21, 28, 29]. Also, return of menses in females with AN is directly associated with weight gain [30]. The weight required for return of menses is highly individual [3, 31, 32]; estimation of treatment goal weight is discussed later in this chapter.

Although weight loss is an important factor affecting the HPO axis and subsequent amenorrhea, research shows that other factors must also be involved. In many patients with AN, amenorrhea precedes significant weight loss [22] suggesting that there are other mechanisms in addition to weight changes involved in the pathogenesis of menstrual abnormalities seen in individuals with AN. Research has also shown that amenorrhea can continue after weight restoration in a proportion of women with AN [33, 34], and that menses can return in some women despite having a low body weight [35, 36].

The Role of Fat Mass

Early research has suggested that there may be a critical amount of body fat required for menarche and for return of menses in patients with AN. In one study, restoration of menstrual cycles occurred at a minimum weight representing 22% body fat [37]; authors hypothesized that a loss of body fat results in a loss of extra-gonadal estrogen and that therefore an increase in body fat contributes to increased estrogen levels as androgens can be aromatized into estrogen in the adipose tissue [37]. In keeping with this theory, women with AN who continue to menstruate have higher fat mass and percent body fat as compared to amenorrheic women with AN [36]. Additionally, women with AN who achieve return of menses, have higher baseline cortisol levels, greater increases in leptin, and greater increases in fat mass than women with AN without return of menses. Increased fat mass predicted menstrual recovery and baseline cortisol levels were associated with increases in percent body fat [38].

The Role of Leptin

Leptin, a hormone made primarily by adipocytes, plays an important role in energy homeostasis. Leptin levels are thought to correlate with body fat [39, 40]; not surprisingly, individuals with AN have low levels of leptin as compared to controls [41] and also as compared to menstruating constitutionally thin women [39]. Although the role of leptin in menstrual function is not completely understood, it is likely that leptin works together with other factors that contribute to menstrual function in AN. Low leptin levels in amenorrhoeic individuals with AN are associated with low LH and estradiol levels [42] and correlated to low IGF-1 levels [39]. One study also found that leptin levels predicted eating-disordered behavior (in addition to fat mass) in underweight patients but also in those who were working towards recovery [43]. Leptin levels remained low in women with AN who are weight restored yet remain amenorrhoeic as compared to those who are weight restored and menstruating [44, 45]. Low levels have also been found in women with purging type eating disorders as compared to non-eating disordered women with similar BMIs [46]. The role of leptin in menstrual dysfunction in AN requires further study.

The Role of Cortisol/Adrenal Function

Cortisol is a glucocorticoid that acts on multiple body systems and reduces LH, estradiol, and progesterone effects. Patients with AN have high levels of serum cortisol as compared to controls, low levels of dehydroepiandrosterone sulfate (DHEAS) but normal levels of adrenocorticotropic hormone (ACTH) [20]. The high level of cortisol is thought to be secondary to excess secretion of corticotropin-releasing hormone (CRH) as well as an over-responsive adrenal gland [20]. Patients who recover from AN and are weight restored appear to have a normalized hypothalamic-pituitary-adrenal axis [47].

The Role of Disordered Eating and Over-Exercise

Disordered eating and intense exercise have both individually been found to affect the menstrual cycle regardless of a woman's absolute weight. For example, weight-recovered amenorrhoeic patients with AN were found to restrict their dietary fat intake whereas weight-recovered patients with AN who had return of their menses did not [48]. Moreover, amenorrhea and oligomenorrhoea can develop in individuals who participate in strenuous exercise, even if their weight is preserved [49]. In non-eating disordered individuals, the mechanism of exercise-induced amenorrhea relates to a decrease in GnRH pulse frequency that results in low levels of gonadotropins and estradiol [50]; interestingly, administration of exogenous GnRH leads to an exaggerated LH secretion response in non-eating disordered athletes with amenorrhea, but leads to normalization of LH secretion in patients with AN with amenorrhea [51]. In a study comparing patients with underweight/low weight eating disorders who were amenorrhoeic and those who were still menstruating, only BMI and intense exercise strongly correlated with amenorrhea [12]. Similarily, Pinheiro et al. found that, in addition to BMI and caloric intake, level of exercise was strongly associated with menstrual status in patients with AN as well as other types of eating disorders [21].

The Role of Psychopathology

It is known that certain psychiatric conditions can affect a woman's menstrual status. Anxiety, depression and stress (which are all commonly seen in individuals with AN) are associated with increased cortisol secretion as well as an inhibition of GnRH secretion, which can then lead to menstrual dysfunction [52]. Additionally, malnutrition and the resultant lack of estrogen affects serotonin function as well as the pathways that regulate cognition and affect [53, 54].

Studies investigating the specific role of patient psychopathology on menstrual dysfunction in AN have generally found that there are few differences in psychopathology between women with AN who menstruate and those who do not menstruate. Several studies have consistently found no differences in prevalence of comorbid psychiatric disorders in menstruating patients with AN versus those who were amenorrheic [9, 12, 21, 29, 55]. Some research, however, has shown that an individual's personality profile may be associated with menstrual status in AN [9, 21]. For example, two studies found that amenorrheic women with AN had lower Temperament and Character inventory (TCI) novelty seeking scores as compared to women with AN and other eating disorders who had normal menstruation or oligomenorrhea [9, 21]. Also, Pinheiro et al. found that women with eating disorders and menstrual dysfunction had higher scores on rituals and obsessions measures as compared to women with eating disorders who had normal menstruation [21]. The relationship between psychopathology and menstrual function in patients with AN needs to be further elucidated.

INVESTIGATIONS

As AN can affect all organ systems of the body, investigations including laboratory tests, electrocardiogram (ECG), bone mineral density are all recommended [5]. Investigations are catered to a patient's individual status depending on the degree of malnutrition, and any abnormal weight control behaviours reported (such as purging, bingeing, laxative use, fasting), in addition to ruling out other potential causes for weight loss (such as hyperthyroidism). A full review of the investigations required in AN is out of the scope of this article and recommendations are published elsewhere [56].

Hormone Tests and Pelvic Ultrasound

In terms of investigations in cases where oligomenorrhoea and amenorrhea are present, hormone levels, including LH, FSH, and estradiol are routinely completed. Pregnancy should be excluded, regardless if weight loss has occurred. In the context of a malnourished, underweight patient with AN, one would expect to see suppressed LH, FSH and estradiol levels and normal prolactin level with usually normal thyroid stimulating hormone (TSH) levels [20]. With weight gain, it is expected that estradiol, LH, FSH levels normalize. Persistent hypoestrogenemia correlates with ongoing ovarian dysfunction and may signal that the patient is not at a healthy weight yet. Previous literature has shown that return of menses is associated with an estradiol level of above 110 pmol/L [30] although clinical practice suggests that this can be variable [32]. Pelvic ultrasonography may also be useful in helping to predict return of menses. As a patient goes from an underweight and hypoestrogenemic state to a weight restored state with spontaneous endogenous estrogen formation, the ovaries shift from a small, amorphous appearance to normal uterine morphology with the appearance of a dominant ovarian follicle; a dominant follicle is defined as one whose growth has accelerated ahead of the other follicles in the same ovary by more than 3 mm and has a diameter of 10 mm or more [57, 58].

Bone Mineral Density Evaluation

In children and adolescents, AN can delay or arrest puberty, which can affect linear growth as well as peak bone mass attainment [24]. As peak bone mass acquisition occurs in the adolescent years and requires endogenous estrogen for optimal development in females, delayed attainment of menarche can lead to a failure to achieve optimal peak bone mass. Additionally, patients with AN are at increased risk for osteopenia and/or osteoporosis which increases the lifetime risk of bone fracture [59].

As the risks to bone are significant, bone mineral density scans are routinely done in patients with AN in order to screen for osteopenia and osteoporosis. Low bone mineral density at all sites is often seen in adolescents with AN, however sites of primarily trabecular bone are preferentially affected [60]. One of the most significant causes of low bone density and decreased bone accrual seen in AN is hypothalamic hypogonadism with low estrogen being an important determinant of low bone mineral density [61]. Other factors involved in decreasing bone density in patients with AN include high cortisol levels, low insulin-like growth factor (IGF-1) levels and variations in leptin [62].

MANAGEMENT

Management of AN requires a multidisciplinary specialized treatment team approach, including medical monitoring, dietetic and nutritional support, and psychological and psychiatric treatment. From a medical point of view, weight restoration is the cornerstone of treatment. Reaching a healthy weight supports proper normal physical growth and development, puberty, as well as optimal psychological functioning [3]. Despite the exclusion of the amenorrhea criteria from the diagnosis of AN, resumption of menstruation remains an important indicator of recovery from the disease [63].

Determination of an Individual Healthy Body Weight

There is a lack of consensus on the method to determine the ideal body weight that an undernourished anorexic patient needs to attain during treatment. Previous practices included using median weights for age on standard growth charts (i.e., 50th percentiles), but current trends increasingly rely on individual characteristics to determine a treatment goal weight range. In adults, the premorbid weight is often used. In pediatric and adolescent patients, it is important to take into account age, premorbid trajectory for height and weight, stage of pubertal development, and growth potential [3, 64]. Additionally, weight goals need to be reassessed frequently in adolescent patients during periods of growth [3]. The treatment goal weight can be a moving target during adolescence depending on the growth potential remaining. It is important to reassess the target weight every 3 – 6 months during periods of growth [3].

In adolescence, pre-pubertal weights can be useful to predict an ideal body weight occurring during puberty, returning to a weight trajectory preceding the weight loss [31, 65]. Previous studies have shown that a weight of approximately 90% standard body weight was the average weight at which resumption of menses occurred [30], although more recent studies have suggested 95% as a minimum of the target weight [65]. If the menstrual threshold weight, or weight at which menses was lost, is known, it has been suggested a weight of 2 kg higher is needed to restore menses [30].

There is good evidence that weight gain and subsequent return of menses (or achievement of menarche) can improve bone mineral density in women with AN [66] and as such, the first line treatment for low bone density in the setting of AN is weight gain [61]. Despite limited research, there is some evidence that the use of bisphosphonates in adult patients can improve BMD [67]; in adolescents, however, bisphosphonates have not been shown to be effective [68]. As it relates to the role of hormone replacement or estrogen therapies (in the oral format), the vast majority of studies in this area have found no benefit of these treatments on bone mineral density [69, 70]. There is some promising research investigating the use of transdermal estrogen patches to help increase bone mineral density in adolescents. Misra and colleagues found that the 17B-estradiol transdermal patch used in girls with a bone age above 15 years, and a small but escalating dose of ethinyl estradiol used in girls with a bone age less than 15 years, improved spine and hip bone mineral density scores as compared to controls [71].

It is also important to consider that spontaneous return of menses can be a helpful marker of an appropriate recovered weight and this must be balanced with any perceived benefit of estrogen treatment, which appears to be limited [20]. Further prospective research is needed in this area to advance our understanding of treatments that serve to improve bone mineral density in this population.

PROGNOSIS

Long-term prognosis of AN varies and can depend on physical, social and psychological factors; low body mass, a greater severity of social and psychological problems, self-induced vomiting and laxative abuse are predictors of poor outcome [72]. One study that followed 84 patients for 21 years after their first hospitalization for AN, found that 50·6% of patients achieved full recovery, 10·4% still met full diagnostic criteria for AN, and 15·6% had died from causes related to AN [73]. Similarily, Steinhausen et al. [74] found that 46% of patients fully recovered from AN, a third improved with only partial features of the disorder, and 20% remained chronically ill for the long term. The standardized mortality ratios (SMRs) of AN reported in the literature vary substantially up to 17.8, with an average of 6.2 (95% CI 5.5–7.0) [19]. The most common causes of death reported are suicide and physical sequelae secondary to the illness, such as cardiovascular complications [19]. In terms of menstrual function and fertility, long term follow up studies have not demonstrated any issues with fertility in women with AN who achieve a healthy weight and return of menses [75, 76].

CONCLUSION

AN is a potentially devastating disease that can affect every organ system. Menstrual function can be affected early in the course of illness, but does not always necessarily correlate with the degree of weight lost. Indeed, patients that are near normal weight may develop amenorrhea and conversely women and youth with significant weight loss may in some cases continue to menstruate. As such, regulated menstrual function can be considered a critical piece of a complex puzzle of health determination in AN that is influenced by a myriad of physiological factors. Early and effective treatment is important to help stave off the pronounced morbidity and high rates of mortality observed in AN. The return of normalized menstrual function in patients with AN and amenorrhea or oligomenorrhea through adequate and maintained weight control should be a priority for health care providers. Although determination of hormone levels as well as the determination of ovarian and uterine markers on pelvic ultrasound may help inform treatment progress, the return of a normalized and regulated menstrual period remains a key indicator of overall health. In cases where patients continue to menstruate despite significant weight loss, health care providers should ensure that other markers of medical health including vital signs are normalized and target persistent and interfering eating disorder behaviors. In cases where amenorrhea persists despite what is perceived as normalized weight, further investigations should be undertaken including reassessment of an individual's calculated target or healthy weight, as well as reassessment of other behaviours that can also affect the menstrual cycle, such as disordered eating or over-exercise. Further research is needed to continue to explore the mechanisms of menstrual dysfunction in AN and its treatment in order to improve outcomes in this population.

REFERENCES

[1] Hoek H. W., van H. D. Review of the prevalence and incidence of eating disorders. *Int. J. Eat Disord.* 34; 383-96.

[2] Hoek H. W. Incidence, prevalence and mortality of anorexia nervosa and other eating disorders. *Curr. Opin. Psychiatry* 19; 389-94.

[3] Golden N. H., Katzman D. K., Sawyer S. M. et al. Update on the medical management of eating disorders in adolescents. *J. Adolesc. Health* 56; 370-5.

[4] American Psychiatric Association Task Force. Diagnostic and statistical manual of mental disorders: DSM-5. Washington, D.C.: *American Psychiatric Association*, 2013.

[5] Katzman D. K. Medical complications in adolescents with anorexia nervosa: a review of the literature. *Int. J. Eat. Disord.* 37 Suppl.; S52-S59.

[6] Franko D. L., Keshaviah A., Eddy K. T. et al. A longitudinal investigation of mortality in anorexia nervosa and bulimia nervosa. *Am. J. Psychiatry* 170; 917-25.

[7] Arcelus J., Mitchell A. J., Wales J., Nielsen S. Mortality rates in patients with anorexia nervosa and other eating disorders. A meta-analysis of 36 studies. *Arch. Gen. Psychiatry* 68; 724-31.

[8] Abraham S. F., Pettigrew B., Boyd C., Russell J., Taylor A. Usefulness of amenorrhea in the diagnoses of eating disorder patients. *J. Psychosom. Obstet. Gynaecol.* 26; 211-5.

[9] Gendall K. A., Joyce P. R., Carter F. A., McIntosh V. V., Jordan J., Bulik C. M. The psychobiology and diagnostic significance of amenorrhea in patients with anorexia nervosa. *Fertil. Steril.* 85; 1531-5.

[10] Roberto C. A., Steinglass J., Mayer L. E., Attia E, Walsh BT The clinical significance of amenorrhea as a diagnostic criterion for anorexia nervosa. *Int. J. Eat. Disord.* 41; 559-63.

[11] Attia E., Roberto C. A. Should amenorrhea be a diagnostic criterion for anorexia nervosa? *Int. J. Eat. Disord.* 42; 581-9.

[12] Dalle G. R., Calugi S, Marchesini G. Is amenorrhea a clinically useful criterion for the diagnosis of anorexia nervosa? *Behav. Res. Ther.* 46; 1290-4.

[13] van Son G. E., van H. D., Bartelds A. I., van Furth E. F., Hoek H. W. Time trends in the incidence of eating disorders: a primary care study in the Netherlands. *Int. J. Eat. Disord.* 39; 565-9.

[14] Favaro A., Caregaro L., Tenconi E., Bosello R., Santonastaso P. Time trends in age at onset of anorexia nervosa and bulimia nervosa. *J. Clin. Psychiatry* 70; 1715-21.

[15] Raevuori A., Keski-Rahkonen A., Hoek H. W. A review of eating disorders in males. *Curr. Opin. Psychiatry* 27; 426-30.

[16] Strother E., Lemberg R., Stanford S. C., Turberville D Eating disorders in men: underdiagnosed, undertreated, and misunderstood. *Eat. Disord.* 20; 346-55.

[17] Rome E. S., Ammerman S. Medical complications of eating disorders: an update. *J. Adolesc. Health* 33; 418-26.

[18] Sullivan P. F. Mortality in anorexia nervosa. *Am. J. Psychiatry* 152; 1073-4.

[19] Papadopoulos F. C., Ekbom A., Brandt L., Ekselius L. Excess mortality, causes of death and prognostic factors in anorexia nervosa. *The British Journal of Psychiatry* 194; 10-7.

[20] Mitan L. A. Menstrual dysfunction in anorexia nervosa. *J. Pediatr. Adolesc. Gynecol.* 17; 81-5.

[21] Poyastro Pinheiro A. a, Thornton L. M., Plotonicov K. H. et al. Patterns of menstrual disturbance in eating disorders. *Int. J. Eat. Disord.* 40; 424-34.

[22] Halmi K. A. Anorexia Nervosa: Demographic and Clinical Features in 94 Cases. *Psychosomatic Medicine* 36.

[23] Mehler P. S., Rylander M Bulimia Nervosa - medical complications. *J. Eat. Disord. 3*; 12.

[24] Vyver E., Steinegger C, Katzman DK Eating disorders and menstrual dysfunction in adolescents. *Ann. N. Y. Acad. Sci.* 1135; 253-64.

[25] Marshall J. C., Kelch R. P. Low dose pulsatile gonadotropin-releasing hormone in anorexia nervosa: a model of human pubertal development. *J. Clin. Endocrinol. Metab.* 49; 712-8.

[26] Boyar R. M., Katz J., Finkelstein J. W. et al. Anorexia nervosa. Immaturity of the 24-hour luteinizing hormone secretory pattern. *N. Engl. J. Med.* 291; 861-5.

[27] Wakeling A., DeSouza V. A., Beardwood C. J. Assessment of the negative and positive feedback effects of administered oestrogen on gonadotrophin release in patients with anorexia nervosa. *Psychol. Med.* 7; 397-405.

[28] Copeland PM, Sacks NR, Herzog DB Longitudinal follow-up of amenorrhea in eating disorders. *Psychosom. Med.* 57; 121-6.

[29] Cachelin F. M., Maher B. A. Is amenorrhea a critical criterion for anorexia nervosa? *J. Psychosom. Res.* 44; 435-40.

[30] Golden N. H., Jacobson M. S., Schebendach J., Solanto M. V., Hertz S. M., Shenker I. R. Resumption of menses in anorexia nervosa. *Arch. Pediatr. Adolesc. Med.* 151; 16-21.

[31] Swenne I. Weight requirements for return of menstruations in teenage girls with eating disorders, weight loss and secondary amenorrhea. *Acta Paediatr.* 93; 1449-55.

[32] Harrison M. E., Obeid N., Fu M. C., Norris M. L. Growth curves in short supply: a descriptive study of the availability and utility of growth curve data in adolescents with eating disorders. *BMC Fam. Pract.* 14; 134.

[33] Falk J. R., Halmi K. A. Amenorrhea in anorexia nervosa: examination of the critical body weight hypothesis. *Biol. Psychiatry* 17; 799-806.

[34] Brambilla F., Monteleone P., Bortolotti F. et al. Persistent amenorrhea in weight-recovered anorexics: psychological and biological aspects. *Psychiatry Res.* 118; 249-57.

[35] Walters E. E., Kendler K. S. Anorexia nervosa and anorexic-like syndromes in a population-based female twin sample. *Am. J. Psychiatry* 152; 64-71.

[36] Miller K. K., Grinspoon S., Gleysteen S. et al. Preservation of neuroendocrine control of reproductive function despite severe undernutrition. *J. Clin. Endocrinol. Metab.* 89; 4434-8.

[37] Frisch R. E., McArthur J. W. Menstrual cycles: fatness as a determinant of minimum weight for height necessary for their maintenance or onset. *Science* 185; 949-51.

[38] Misra M., Prabhakaran R., Miller K. K. et al. Role of cortisol in menstrual recovery in adolescent girls with anorexia nervosa. *Pediatr. Res.* 59; 598-603.

[39] Di C. C., Tommaselli G. A., De F. E. et al. Menstrual status and serum leptin levels in anorectic and in menstruating women with low body mass indexes. *Fertil. Steril.* 78; 376-82.

[40] Matejek N., Weimann E., Witzel C., Molenkamp G., Schwidergall S., Bohles H Hypoleptinaemia in patients with anorexia nervosa and in elite gymnasts with anorexia athletica. *Int. J. Sports Med.* 20; 451-6.

[41] Mehler P. S., Eckel R. H., Donahoo W. T. Leptin levels in restricting and purging anorectics. *Int. J. Eat. Disord.* 26; 189-94.

[42] Hebebrand J., Muller T. D., Holtkamp K., Herpertz-Dahlmann B. The role of leptin in anorexia nervosa: clinical implications. *Mol. Psychiatry* 12; 23-35.

[43] Nakai Y., Hamagaki S., Kato S., Seino Y., Takagi R, Kurimoto F. Role of leptin in women with eating disorders. *Int. J. Eat. Disord.* 26; 29-35.

[44] Misra M., Miller K. K., Almazan C. et al. Hormonal and body composition predictors of soluble leptin receptor, leptin, and free leptin index in adolescent girls with anorexia nervosa and controls and relation to insulin sensitivity. *J. Clin. Endocrinol. Metab.* 89; 3486-95.

[45] Katzman D. K., Golden N. H., Neumark-Sztainer D., Yager J., Strober M. From prevention to prognosis: clinical research update on adolescent eating disorders. *Pediatr. Res.* 47; 709-12.

[46] Jimerson D. C., Wolfe B. E., Carroll DP, Keel PK Psychobiology of purging disorder: reduction in circulating leptin levels in purging disorder in comparison with controls. *Int. J. Eat. Disord.* 43; 584-8.

[47] Gold P. W., Gwirtsman H., Avgerinos PC et al. Abnormal hypothalamic-pituitary-adrenal function in anorexia nervosa. Pathophysiologic mechanisms in underweight and weight-corrected patients. *N. Engl. J. Med.* 314; 1335-42.

[48] Couzinet B., Young J., Brailly S., Le B. Y., Chanson P, Schaison G. Functional hypothalamic amenorrhea: a partial and reversible gonadotrophin deficiency of nutritional origin. *Clin. Endocrinol.* (Oxf) 50; 229-35.

[49] Bullen B. A., Skrinar G. S., Beitins I. Z., von M. G., Turnbull B. A., McArthur J. W. Induction of menstrual disorders by strenuous exercise in untrained women. *N. Engl. J. Med.* 312; 1349-53.

[50] Kazis K., Iglesias E. The female athlete triad. *Adolesc. Med.* 14; 87-95.

[51] Golden N. H., Shenker I. R. Amenorrhea in anorexia nervosa. Neuroendocrine control of hypothalamic dysfunction. *Int. J. Eat. Disord.* 16; 53-60.

[52] Young E. A., Korszun A. The hypothalamic-pituitary-gonadal axis in mood disorders. *Endocrinol. Metab. Clin. North Am.* 31; 63-78.

[53] Rubinow DR, Schmidt PJ, Roca CA Estrogen-serotonin interactions: implications for affective regulation. *Biol. Psychiatry* 44; 839-50.

[54] McEwen B. Estrogen actions throughout the brain. Recent Prog Horm Res 57; 357-84.

[55] Kreipe R. E., Strauss J, Hodgman C. H., Ryan R. M. Menstrual cycle abnormalities and subclinical eating disorders: a preliminary report. *Psychosom. Med.* 51; 81-6.

[56] Pritts S. D., Susman J Diagnosis of eating disorders in primary care. *Am. Fam. Physician* 67; 297-304.

[57] Treasure J. L., Wheeler M., King E. A., Gordon P. A., Russell GF Weight gain and reproductive function: ultrasonographic and endocrine features in anorexia nervosa. *Clin. Endocrinol.* (Oxf) 29; 607-16.

[58] Treasure J. L. The ultrasonographic features in anorexia nervosa and bulimia nervosa: a simplified method of monitoring hormonal states during weight gain. *J. Psychosom. Res.* 32; 623-34.

[59] Misra M., Klibanski A. Anorexia nervosa and osteoporosis. *Rev. Endocr. Metab. Disord.* 7; 91-9.

[60] Misra M., Aggarwal A., Miller K. K. et al. Effects of anorexia nervosa on clinical, hematologic, biochemical, and bone density parameters in community-dwelling adolescent girls. *Pediatrics* 114; 1574-83.

[61] Katzman D. K., Misra M. Bone health in adolescent females with anorexia nervosa: what is a clinician to do? *Int. J. Eat. Disord.* 46; 456-60.

[62] Misra M., Klibanski A. Bone health in anorexia nervosa. *Curr. Opin. Endocrinol. Diabetes Obes.* 18; 376-82.

[63] Couturier J., Lock J. What is recovery in adolescent anorexia nervosa? *Int. J. Eat. Disord.* 39; 550-5.

[64] Golden N. H., Jacobson M. S., Sterling W. M., Hertz S. Treatment goal weight in adolescents with anorexia nervosa: use of BMI percentiles. *Int. J. Eat. Disord.* 41; 301-6.

[65] Faust J. P., Goldschmidt AB, Anderson K. E. et al. Resumption of menses in anorexia nervosa during a course of family-based treatment. *J. Eat. Disord.* 1; 12.

[66] Misra M., Prabhakaran R., Miller K. K. et al. Weight gain and restoration of menses as predictors of bone mineral density change in adolescent girls with anorexia nervosa-1. *J. Clin. Endocrinol. Metab.* 93; 1231-7.

[67] Miller K. K., Meenaghan E., Lawson E. A. et al. Effects of risedronate and low-dose transdermal testosterone on bone mineral density in women with anorexia nervosa: a randomized, placebo-controlled study. *J. Clin. Endocrinol. Metab.* 96; 2081-8.

[68] Golden N. H., Iglesias E. A., Jacobson M. S. et al. Alendronate for the treatment of osteopenia in anorexia nervosa: a randomized, double-blind, placebo-controlled trial. *J. Clin. Endocrinol. Metab.* 90; 3179-85.

[69] Lebow J., Sim L. The influence of estrogen therapies on bone mineral density in premenopausal women with anorexia nervosa and amenorrhea. *Vitam. Horm.* 92; 243-57.

[70] Sim L. A., McGovern L., Elamin M. B., Swiglo B. A., Erwin P. J., Montori V. M. Effect on bone health of estrogen preparations in premenopausal women with anorexia nervosa: a systematic review and meta-analyses. *Int. J. Eat. Disord.* 43; 218-25.

[71] Misra M., Katzman D., Miller K. K. et al. Physiologic estrogen replacement increases bone density in adolescent girls with anorexia nervosa. *J. Bone Miner. Res. 26*; 2430-8.

[72] Lowe B., Zipfel S., Buchholz C., Dupont Y., Reas D. L., Herzog W. Long-term outcome of anorexia nervosa in a prospective 21-year follow-up study. *Psychol. Med.* 31; 881-90.

[73] Zipfel S., Lowe B., Reas D. L., Deter H. C., Herzog W Long-term prognosis in anorexia nervosa: lessons from a 21-year follow-up study. *Lancet* 355; 721-2.

[74] Steinhausen H. C. Outcome of eating disorders. *Child Adolesc. Psychiatr. Clin. N. Am.* 18; 225-42.

[75] Kreipe R. E., Churchill BH, Strauss J Long-term outcome of adolescents with anorexia nervosa. *Am. J. Dis. Child* 143; 1322-7.

[76] Katz M. G., Vollenhoven B. The reproductive endocrine consequences of anorexia nervosa. *BJOG* 107; 707-13.

In: Amenorrhea
Editor: Oliver Chukwujekwu Ezechi
ISBN: 978-1-63484-778-0

Chapter 17

MENSTRUAL IRREGULARITIES IN OBESITY

George Uchenna Eleje[1] and Victor O. Oboro[2]
[1]Department of Obstetrics and Gynaecology, Faculty of Medicine, College of Health Sciences, Nnamdi Azikiwe University, Nnewi, Nigeria
[2]Department of Obstetrics and Gynaecology, Ladoke Akintola University of Technology, Ogbomosho, Nigeria

ABSTRACT

Obesity remains a common and global problem in women of reproductive age. It involves an abnormal and disproportionate body fat accumulation that negatively affects menstrual function. The World Health Organization defined obesity as body mass index equals to or greater than 30 kg/m^2. Its prevalence is increasing worldwide and obese women have been shown to have a higher incidence of menstrual dysfunction. The International Obesity Task Force reported that 312 million adults are obese. The risks for menstrual abnormalities are increased many fold by increase in truncal obesity. Several proposed mechanisms explain how obesity leads to menstrual abnormalities; however, the exact pathophysiology remains unclear. It is thought that the menstrual irregularity in obesity is mainly hormone mediated. Leptin levels are increased in obese women with stimulatory effect on the hypothalamo-pituitary-ovarian axis. Treatment remains weight reduction and certain pharmacological agents. However, it is difficult to treat menstrual abnormalities in obese women since they require a higher dosage of drug therapy, hence poor response to menstrual regulation is predominant. The first line management of menstrual irregularity in obese women is weight loss. The first weight loss goal should be to halt further weight gain and stay at the current level, since this would cut their risk of obesity-related complications by a disproportionate 50%. The ultimate goal, however, is to lose more than 15 percent of body weight and maintaining same, rather than achieving an 'ideal' weight.

Keywords: obesity, menstrual irregularities, weight loss, overweight

INTRODUCTION

Obesity remains a common problem among women of reproductive age. It involves an abnormal and excessive body fat accumulation that negatively affects the health of the body. The World Health Organization (WHO) defines obesity as the body mass index (BMI) equal to or greater than 30 kg/m^2, and overweight as BMI of 25 to 29.9 kg/m^2 (Table 1) [1-3].

Obesity has become a world-wide pandemic in the last 20 years. It is estimated that the prevalence of overweight and obesity has more than doubled from 1980 to 2000.

Current estimate suggests that about a third of US population is obese, with 5% of the population being extremely obese [2]. The figures also show that around two-thirds of the American adult population is either overweight or obese, with the rate for childhood obesity being around 20%, a four-fold increase from 1970. According to the World Health Organization in 2003, obesity is one of the most serious world health problems. The consequences of obesity are wide ranging, and include reproductive health problems [3].

In women, obesity plays a noteworthy part in reproductive tract abnormalities. It is often associated with anovulation and menstrual disorders. Additionally, obesity is associated with anovulatory infertility, difficulties in assisted reproduction and several pregnancy and fetal complications (Table 2).

Obesity is associated with several pregnancy and fetal complications (Table 2), Obesity is also associated with anovulatory infertility, and it is estimated that about 4% decline in fecundity occur for every BMI values in excess of 29 kg/m^2. On the other hand, weight loss has been shown to improve fertility, and success following *In-vitro* fertilization is higher in the lower BMI categories. Miscarriage rate is also increased in obese women, and as part of contemporary fertility management it is recommended that treatment be delayed until some degree of weight loss has been achieved for overweight and obese women [4].

EPIDEMIOLOGY AND PREDISPOSING FACTORS OF OBESITY

Overweight represent a rapidly growing threat to the health of populations and an increasing number of countries globally. Excess bodyweight is now the sixth most important risk factor contributing to the overall burden of disease worldwide. Over 1·1 billion adults and 10% of children globally are now classified as overweight or obese [5]. Obesity has increased in developed countries because of a more sedentary lifestyle, including reduced physical activity, changes in nutrition style, and an increased calorie intake. However, some other factors such as genetic, disorders of endocrine, hormones, and psychological, including the use of some drugs such as steroids and antidepressants may lead to obesity [4, 5]. Possibly ethnic factors may prove to be important in determining the magnitude of the complications associated with obesity.

Table 1. Classification of Obesity

Body mass index	Classification
Underweight	<18.5
Normal range	18.5-24.9
Overweight	≥25
Preobese	25.0-29.9
Obese class I	30.0-34.9
Obese class II	35.0-39.9
Obese class III	≥40

Table 2. Pregnancy and fetal complications of obesity

Pregnancy	Fetal
Pre-eclampsia	Fetal cardiac defect
Hypertension	Neural birth defects
Impaired glucose tolerance	Macrosomia
Gestational diabetes	Shoulder dystocia
Operative delivery	

Table 3. Adverse reproductive outcome in obese women

Adverse outcome
1. Precocious menarche
2. Menstrual irregularities
3. Chronic anovulation
4. Increased risk of miscarriage
5. Decreased conception rates after assisted reproductive technologies
6. Increased morbidity in pregnant women
7. Worsened outcomes of preterm deliveries
8. Increased androgenisation

Obesity and Reproductive Health of Women

Women who are overweight or obese have been shown to have higher incidence of poor reproductive health outcome compared to those who are of normal body mass index. With the rising prevalence of overweight and obesity worldwide, it is of utmost importance to consider these effects on women's reproductive health. Increasingly significant associations have been reported between excess body fat and irregular menstrual cycles, reduced spontaneous and induced fertility, increased risk of miscarriage and hormone-sensitive carcinomas (Table 3). The observed abnormalities have been attributed to changes in circulating sex hormones.

The type of obesity might influence the association with reproductive outcome including menstrual irregularity. Centrally distributed body fat has been shown to have stronger association with abnormal hormonal profile and irregular menstrual pattern than peripherally distributed or overall adiposity. Abnormal uterine bleeding occurred three times more frequently in women with upper body fat predominance compared with women with lower body fat predominance.

Pathophysiology

The mechanism by which obesity results in menstrual irregularity is probably hormone mediated. It has been demonstrated that the levels of testosterone, total and free, is increased (along with a corresponding decrease in level of sex hormone-binding globulin (SHBG) in women with obesity, central or otherwise [6]. There is a positive dose-response curve for the relationship between testosterone concentration and body fat composition and polycystic ovary syndrome, the latter is associated with abnormal uterine bleeding, anovulation and infertility related to the ovulatory dysfunction and menstrual irregularity. In another study the free androgen index (FAI), which is a measure of testosterone in relation to SHBG actually has a stronger effect on menstrual irregularity than testosterone alone, suggesting that SHBG is more important in the causal association between overweight/obesity and irregular menstruation. The SHBG itself is affected by the level of the glucose regulatory hormone insulin. Indeed, when adjusted for the effect of SHBG, FAI, and insulin, there was a substantial attenuation in the association between overweight/obesity and menstrual irregularity [6].

Obesity and Menstrual Abnormality

Adipose tissues are capable of making a weak estrogen, estrone, and releasing it into the circulation. Although weaker than estradiol, it is capable of suppressing follicle stimulating hormone (FSH) release and preventing the full development of a dominant follicle. When this occurs, developing follicles will progress to about 10 mm in size, add estradiol to the circulating pool of hormones, and be unable to grow further due to the decreasing levels of FSH occurring secondary to the negative feedback estrogens exert on FSH excretion. The ovaries will therefore obtain a "polycystic appearance" due to the many small follicles present at the periphery which are unable to fully develop with the falling FSH levels. Androgen levels rise with the falling FSH levels since FSH stimulates the aromatization of androgens to estrogens. A high androgen environment within the developing follicle leads to follicular atresia. The resulting elevated serum androgens exert an inhibitory effect on hepatic protein production, which leads to decreased production of SHBG. SHBG binds estrogens and androgens in the serum making them less active. With less SHBG, the amount of free testosterone in the serum increases causing further atresia and hirsutism.

Additionally, some patients with obesity have insulin resistance, a condition where their cells do not respond adequately to insulin so they must maintain elevated serum insulin levels in order to regulate glucose. One theory for this disorder is an insulin receptor defect. Insulin is capable of activating the IGF-II receptor and stimulating the theca cells to produce excess amounts of androgens leading to PCOS. Therefore, patients with insulin resistance can develop PCOS and subsequent menstrual abnormality.

Anovulation and Menstrual Disturbances

The mechanism of anovulation in obesity remains unclear. However, attention currently is focused on 1) Disturbed estrogen metabolism, 2) decreased sex hormone-binding globulin, 3) insulin resistance and hyper insulinemia and 4) leptin abnormality.

Insulin resistance and hyperandrogenemia are significantly increased in obese women, particularly in women with central obesity. Hyperandrogenemia due to hyperinsulinemia leads to granulosa cell apoptosis, and this may have an effect on ovarian functions.

The effect of FSH on estradiol and progesterone production is increased by insulin. This is demonstrated in women with PCOS and insulin resistance. Thus, the estrogen level increases in the developing follicle. FSH enhances the excessive androgen substrate, leading to relatively improper estrogen levels in the developing follicle. Insulin also enhances steroidogenesis by augmenting the effect of luitenising hormone (LH) on granulosa cells. LH stimulates steroidogenesis and inhibits further mitosis and final differentiation of granulosa cells in the preovulatory follicle [7]. The effect of LH on granulosa cells is amplified in PCOS patients by the presence of hyperinsulinemia.

As a result of the enhanced steroidogenesis due to insulin and its interaction with LH, the unfavorable milieu causes cessation of the follicle growth. Thus, premature luteinization and follicular arrest develops and leads to menstrual cycle disorders and obesity-induced oligoanovulation [8]. A characteristic feature of the blood hormone profile in obese women is high levels of androgen and LH. Obese individual may have insulin resistance and hyperinsulinemia. This leads to thickening of the theca cell layer in the ovaries and results in increased production of androgen in the ovary. In addition, hyperinsulinemia induces a decrease in SHBG in the liver, and decreased SHBG may further increase active androgen, influencing ovulation and menstrual cycle. The increased estrogen due to peripheral conversion disturbs the HPG axis. The excess estrogen and excess androgens thus play a role in the anovulation encountered in these patients.

Large fat cells produce correspondingly large estrogens, which cause the body to react as if in case of contraception. In obese, adipocytes secret adipokines (leptin, adiponectin, omentin, resistin, ghrelin and visfatin), which have important roles in the regulation of a number of physiological processes including menstruation. Leptin levels are increased in obese and this has a stimulatory effect on the hypothalamo-pituitary-ovarian axis. The observation that leptin-deficient obese mice were infertile, but regained fertility following leptin supplementation, has focused attention on leptin as a possible cause of menstrual disorder in obese women [9].

Several studies have shown that obese women are more likely to experience menstrual cycle irregularity than non-obese women [7-9].

Menstrual Cycle Related Changes in Appetite

Appetite or food intake undergoes significant changes in response to the menstrual cycle. Several studies have shown that that food intake is reduced around the time of ovulation but increased in the luteal phase of the menstrual cycle in primates [10]. Similarly, increased food intake has been shown to be increased premenstrually in women with premenstrual dysphoric syndrome. This appetite changes thus corresponds with ovarian hormone changes, implying that estrogen, which surges during ovulation, suppresses appetite, while progesterone (highest in the luteal or premenstrual phase) stimulates the appetite to promote food intake.

MANAGEMENT

Diagnosis

Obesity or overweight as a cause of menstrual irregularity is a diagnosis of exclusion. All the other causes of menstrual irregularities should been excluded before it is attributed to overweight/obesity. Tests of ovulation and hormone profile are often performed as part of management of menstrual irregularities. The hormonal pattern in obesity or overweight may overlap with those of Polycystic Ovarian Diseases or other endocrinopathies, with anovulatory cycles occurring as part of menstrual irregularities.

Treatment

Irrespective of whether or not ovulatory dysfunction or hormonal imbalance is identified, menstrual irregularity in the context of overweight and obesity should be managed as first line approach.

Weight loss is the first step in the management of menstrual irregularity in obese patient, and only when this fails is further treatment generally advocated. Although distribution of adiposity features prominently in the frequency of menstrual irregularity, it is conventional to offer weight loss as the first step in the management of the menstrual irregularity irrespective of whether obesity is central or peripheral in distribution. It is also important that the weight-hip ratio or Trung-Leg Ratio, should not influence whether or not weight loss is recommended for anyone whose BMI is 30 or above [11, 12].

The treatment options for overweight and obesity are based on the medical history, and may include combination of options, ranging from lifestyle modifications, diet and exercise, medication and surgery. But it should all start with setting weight loss goal that is realistic, with the understanding that drastic weight loss could actually be detrimental to health. The goal is to reduce the health consequences of overweight and obesity, and as such the return of regular menstrual pattern can be used as a good gauge of weight loss success. A first weight loss goal should be to halt further weight gain and stay at the current level (within, for example, 5% or 5 pounds). It has been shown that those at a high risk for developing diabetes would, by losing a mere 5% of their body weight, would cut their risk of developing diabetes by a disproportionate 50%, reduce their blood pressure and achieve a regular menstrual pattern. The ultimate goal is to lose more than 15 percent of body weight and maintaining same, rather than achieving an 'ideal' weight [11, 12].

Lifestyle Changes

The main goals in lifestyle changes include modifying eating habits, being more active, and making healthier choices relating to diet and exercise. The goals of lifestyle changes are to help you change your eating habits, become more active, and be more aware of how much you eat and exercise, helping you to make healthier choices. It also involves figuring out triggers to eat, breaking the chain of events between the triggers and the eating, changing the type of diet eating regularly, and practicing positive reinforcement on successful lifestyle modification [12].

Diet

The goal of dietary modification is to reduce the caloric intake below the caloric expenditure. There are many factors affecting energy expenditure, including age, gender and weight. For example, younger people have a more rapid metabolism compared to the older ones, hence they lose weight faster. Similarly, men lose more weight for a given calorie intake than women of same age, height and weight when dieting. Moreover, people who are morbidly obese lose weight more rapidly than those who are just overweight [11, 12].

Dieting involves calculation of daily calorie need based on current weight, gender and activity level. Then food are chosen that contains adequate protein, carbohydrates, essential fatty acids and vitamins, while avoiding alcohol, extra sugar, sweets (cookies, cakes and candy). Because of the calculations involved in determination of calorie and contents of meals, the concept of 'portion-controlled diets' have evolved to simplify dieting. This involves resorting to pre-packaged foods, such as frozen low-calorie meals, meal-replacement drinks or bars. These are then taken thrice a day, for example: a breakfast bar is taken in the morning, a meal-replacement drink as lunch, and a frozen low-calorie (250-350 calorie) meal in combination with extra vegetable for dinner, for a total daily intake of 1000-1500 calories in a day.

If the trouble can be taken to estimate the content of meals, then the following guidelines are helpful. For fat estimates, a low-fat diet is one in which less than 30% of calories are derived from fat. Thus for a daily 1500 calorie diet, this would amount to less than 45 g (based on the calculation that 1 g of fat provides 33.3 calories of energy). For carbohydrate estimation, Low carbohydrate diets, such as Atkins diet, are popular dieting meals. A low carbohydrate diet provides 60-130 g of carbohydrate in a day, while a very-low-carbohydrate diet gives between 0-60 g of carbohydrates per day. This is against the 200-300 g of carbohydrate present in a standard diet. Very-low-carbohydrate diets do result in side effects, such as constipation, diarrhea, bad breath, headache, muscle cramps, and weakness [11, 12].

The Mediterranean diet is another dietary modification method. The Mediterranean diet is based on the traditional foods of people who lived around the Mediterranean Sea egg Italy and Greece in the year 1960. It was observed that these people were exceptionally healthy compared to Americans and a much lower risk of obesity-related complications. The adoption of the Mediterranean diet has been shown in numerous studies to be an effective weight loss measure and prevention of morbidity associated with overweight/obesity. The bases of the diet are:

1. A high amount of monounsaturated fats (egg olive or canola oil, pecans, walnuts and almonds), fruits, vegetables, grains and legumes (7-10 servings of fruits and vegetables per day).
2. A moderate amount of milk and dairy products, largely as cheese, or low-fat dairy products (skim milk, low-fat cheese, fat-free yogurt).
3. A low amount of red meat or meat products (fish or poultry are substituted for red meat) and sweets/simple sugars.

Medications

When used in combination with lifestyle changes, diet and exercise, medication are sometimes helpful in weight loss. However, they are associated with side effects, and therefore the risk-benefit ratio must be taken into consideration. Their main indications are 1) Body mass index (BMI) of 30 or more, BMI of 27-30 with co-morbid illnesses like hypertension, diabetes, or hypercholesterolemia, and 3) where diet, exercise and lifestyle changes have been ineffective.

Wight loss medication options are discussed below.

1. Orlistat — prevents fat absorption in the gastrointestinal system. It is taken thrice daily with meal, but may be omitted if meal is fat-free. If used daily for one year, a weight loss of up to 5 kg may be achieved, or close to 10% of initial body weight may be lost, compared to 4% in those who used placebos. It is also associated with reduction in the risk of obesity-related complications such as hypercholesterolemia, hypertension and diabetes. Side-effects are related to excess fat in stool, and include stomach cramps, diarrhea, gas, leakage of stool, or steatorrhea. They occur in about 10-15% of patients taking the medication, but may increase if meals are high in fat content, or if more than 30% of calories in the diet are derived from fat, thus the side effects could be avoided by avoidance of fatty meals.
2. Lorcaserin — Lorcaserin is an appetite suppressant with similar efficacy to orlistat. Side effects include headache, upper respiratory infections, nasopharyngitis, dizziness, and nausea. It is taken twice daily and contraindicated in renal failure or pregnancy. It is also associated with, serotonin syndrome' if used with serotonergic drugs.
3. Phentermine-extended release topiramate — Phentermine causes early satiety, thereby reducing caloric intake. The mechanism of action of Topiramate, however, is unclear, and its use for the prevention of migraine was associated with weight loss hence its use for that purpose. The medication must be used in a gradually increasing dosage, and it can precipitate seizure if abruptly withdrawn. Pregnancy test is also required before starting the medication, as, like other antiepileptics, it is associated with orofacial clefts in infants who were exposed to the medication. Common side effects include dry mouth, constipation, paraesthesia, psychiatric (depression and anxiety) and cognitive (attention-deficit) disorders. Phentermine-topiramate is used for postmenopausal women or men without cardiovascular disease, especially those who may be intolerant of orlistat or lorcaserin.
4. Bupropion-naltrexone — Bupropion is an antidepressant used to prevent weight gain during smoking-cessation programmes. Naloxone, on the other hand, is used to treat opiate dependence. The combination has similar efficacy as lorcaserine, but more side effects, including nausea/vomiting, headache, constipation, insomnia, dizziness, and dry mouth. It is contraindicated in hypertension, eating disorders, seizure disorders and intake of opioids or monoamine-oxidase inhibitors.
5. Liraglutide — Liraglutide is an antidiabetic with weight loss side effect. Taken at its highest dose can result in weight loss of 7 kg in 6 months, but side effects such as nausea, occurring in 37-47% of cases, vomiting, diarrhea, hypoglycemia and even

pancreatitis, gallbladder disorders, renal disorders and suicidal ideations are present. It is administered subcutaneously.

Weight Loss Surgery [11]

Weight loss surgery (bariatric surgery) is suggested for patients with a BMI ≥40 kg/m^2 in whom diet, exercise and medication have failed to result in significant weight loss. In addition, patients with a BMI >35 kg/m^2 with obesity-related comorbidities (hypertension, diabetes mellitus, hypercholesterolamia, sleep apnea) who have not responded to diet, exercise, and medication are good candidate for bariatric surgery, especially where the anticipated benefit outweighs the risk.

There are different surgical approaches to management of obesity, and available evidence suggests that there is greater weight loss (mean difference - 26 kg) when bariatric surgery is compared to non-surgical treatment of obesity (diet, exercise, weight reducing drugs, behavioral therapy). The weight loss is accompanied by remission in obesity-related complications, but the risks of bariatric surgery should be taken into account in assessing morbidity benefits. Moreover, most trials on surgical management of obesity have been limited by confounding factors such as demographic differences among the population studied, as well as small sample size and short follow-up period. Thus long-term benefits in terms of need for reoperation is yet to be evaluated extensively, but some studies have reported that some weight regain generally occur within three years of surgery. The most frequent risk of bariatric surgery were iron deficiency anemia and the need for reoperations in the short-term, while long-term concerns relates to cardiovascular diseases, diabetic microangiopathies and mortality. Moreover, different surgical modalities have varying success rate in achieving weight reduction. The two main surgical approaches are liposuction and vagal blockade.

Liposuction is fat removal by the process of aspiration after injection of normal saline into the subcutaneous tissue. It can result in significant reduction in weight, but it has not shown promise in improving insulin sensitivity or modify risk factors for ischaemic heart disease. — Removal of fat by aspiration after injection of physiologic saline has been used to remove and contour subcutaneous fat. While this can result in a significant reduction in fat mass and weight, it does not appear to improve insulin sensitivity or risk factors for coronary heart disease.

Vagal blockade — This involves laparoscopic implantation of a device that sends electrical pulses intermittently to abdominal vagal nerve, thus signaling the satiety centre in the brain. This has shown a modest effect on weight loss compared with other bariatric surgeries, but efficacy and safety data are few and there is lack of long-term data to justify its routine use in clinical practice.

CONCLUSION

Obesity is common among women and continue to exert an intense effect on the menstrual function of women, mediated primarily through the endocrine system on multiple levels. Weight loss is the treatment of choice to restore the natural balance to these systems.

When weight loss does not occur, oral contraceptives, progestins, and medications that regulate menstruation can be utilized.

All health programs should emphasize weight loss and exercise for overweight women. This will improve menstrual regularity. In addition, the potential for long-term complications such as diabetes mellitus and cardiovascular disease will be reduced. It is tempting for both physicians and patients to resort immediately to medical treatment such as ovulation induction with gonadotropins or clomiphene citrate, since these measures may not confer long-term benefits to these women. The ultimate goal of management is to lose about 15% of body weight and maintaining same, rather than achieving an 'ideal' weight.

REFERENCES

[1] Rogers, J, Mitchell G. W. The relation of obesity to menstrual disturbances. *New England Journal of Medicine*, 1952;247(2), 53-55.

[2] Flegal, K. M., Carroll, M. D., Kuczmarski, R. J, Johnson, C. L. Overweight and obesity in the United States: prevalence and trends, 1960-1994. *International journal of obesity and related metabolic disorders: journal of the International Association for the Study of Obesity*, 1998;22(1), 39-47.

[3] James, W. P. T. WHO recognition of the global obesity epidemic. *International Journal of Obesity*, 2008;32, S120-S126.

[4] Clark, A. M., Thornley, B., Tomlinson, L., Galletley, C., and Norman, R. J. Weight loss in obese infertile women results in improvement in reproductive outcome for all forms of fertility treatment. *Human Reproduction*, 1998;13(6), 1502-1505.

[5] Haslam, D. W, James, WPT. Obesity. *The Lancet*, 2005;366(9492), 1197-1209.

[6] Glass, A. R., Dahms, W., Abraham, G., Atkinson, R. L., Bray, G. A., werdloff, R. S. Secondary amenorrhea in obesity: etiologic role of weight-related androgen excess. *Fertility and sterility*, 1978;30(2), 243-244.

[7] Hillier SG. Current concepts of the roles of follicle stimulating hormone and luteinizing hormone in folliculogenesis. *Hum Reprod.* 1994;9:188-91.

[8] Franks S, Robinson S, Willis D. Nutrition, insulin and polycistic ovary syndrome. *Rev Reprod.* 1996;1:47-53.

[9] Chapman IM, Wittert GA, Norman RJ. Circulating leptin concentrations in polycystic ovary syndrome: relation to anthropometric and metabolic parameters. *Clin Endocrinol* (Oxf). 1997;46(2):175-81.

[10] Dye, L., Blundell, J. E. Menstrual cycle and appetite control: implications for weight regulation. *Human reproduction*, 1997; 12(6), 1142-1151.

[11] Snow, V., Barry, P., Fitterman, N., Qaseem, A., and Weiss, K. Pharmacologic and surgical management of obesity in primary care: a clinical practice guideline from the American College of Physicians. *Annals of Internal Medicine*, 2005;142(7), 525-531.

[12] O'Brien, S. H., Holubkov, R., Reis, E. C. Identification, evaluation, and management of obesity in an academic primary care center. *Pediatrics*, 2005;114(2), e154-e159.

In: Amenorrhea
Editor: Oliver Chukwujekwu Ezechi

ISBN: 978-1-63484-778-0

Chapter 18

Polycystic Ovarian Disease

Aigbe Gregory Ohihoin
Division of Clinical Sciences, Nigerian Institute of Medical Research, Lagos, Nigeria

Abstract

Polycystic ovarian disease (PCOD) has been described as a condition of chronic anovulation associated with hyperandrogenism. It is the commonest cause of anovulation and hirsutism. The condition is highly heterogeneous and has a broad based symptomatic manifestation that incorporates metabolic dysfunction. The aetiology of PCOD has not been well characterized. Researchers have postulated a genetic basis for the disease, due to its strong association among families. An autosomal dominant pattern has been suggested. In polycystic ovarian disease, there may be no manifestation of symptoms. When symptoms exist, they may manifest as menstrual irregularities, weight gain, hirsutism and infertility. Apart from its gynaecological challenges, PCOD could also have obstetric and medical implications. Patients with PCOD, carry an increased risk of endometrial hyperplasia and invariably greater risk of endometrial carcinoma. The risk of pregnancy losses is higher in women with PCOD. Other obstetric complications linked with PCOD include higher risk of gestational hypertension, gestational diabetes mellitus (GDM), preterm birth and perinatal deaths not linked to multiple gestation.

The laboratory findings will manifest as elevated luteinizing hormone level, normal or low FSH, reduced levels of SHBG, elevated testosterone, hyperinsulinaemia and features of insulin resistance. There could also be laboratory features of metabolic syndrome, manifesting as dyslipidaemia. Diagnosis is made from clinical, biochemical and ultrasonic features. The American Society of Reproductive Medicine (ASRM) and the European Society of Human Reproduction and Embryology (ESHRE) have outlined a set of criteria for the diagnosis of polycystic ovarian disease that consist of having two of the following features: -oligomenorrhoea and or anovulation; clinical and biochemical features of hyperandogenism, and ultrasound features of polycystic ovaries.

The management of patients with PCOD should be tailored to the symptomatology and the individual needs of the woman. The age and reason for presentation will influence management modalities. Careful counselling and follow up may be all that is required in some individuals. Weight loss and exercise programmes can improve symptomatology, menstrual regulation and fertility outcome. The use of oral contraceptive pills (OCPs) and cyclic progestins to regularize menstrual flow has shown good results. Ovulation induction agents such as clomiphene citrate offer a good option for the management of anovulatory infertility. Some workers have suggested the inclusion of insulin sensitizing agents in the armamentarium of therapeutic agents for PCOD. Hirsutism can be managed by pharmacological and mechanical means. Laparoscopic ovarian drilling is a useful adjunct in patients with anovulation unresponsive to ovulation induction agents

Keywords: polycystic ovarian diseases, amenorrhea, menstrual irregularity, insulin resistance, hyperandrogenism

INTRODUCTION

Polycystic ovarian disease (PCOD) is a complex endocrine disorder with diverse metabolic, reproductive and mental health manifestations, with chronic anovolution and hyperadrogenism at the heart of its pathophysiology. PCOD is the commonest endocrine disorder of women of the reproductive age group. The diverse manifestations of polycystic ovarian disease means that there is a broad range of clinicians who will be confronted with the challenge of managing patients with polycystic ovarian disease. The implication of this is that every clinician should have an understanding of the pathophysiology, pattern of presentation and management of the disease.

The true incidence of PCOD has been difficult to establish due to variations in diagnostic criteria over the years. The harmonization of diagnostic criteria by major bodies in reproductive endocrinology has helped to establish some consistency in the determination of its true incidence [1]. The current reported incidence of PCOD is put at about 12-18% of women of the reproductive age [2]. This incidence is based upon criteria from the Rotterdam consensus of 2003 [3]. A higher incidence is documented among women seeking fertility care and in relatively obese population.

Until recently, an understanding of its pathophysiology has been poor, thus it was difficult to determine aetiological factors.

Patients with polycystic ovarian disease should be under clinical surveillance and follow up all through life because they may manifest other features of metabolic dysfunction later in life after the reproductive age has elapsed [4].

EPIDEMIOLOGY

The aetiological factors involved in polycystic ovarian disease have been poorly understood for many years, and this forms the basis of the challenge it poses to clinicians in the management of this condition. Genetic models have been postulated, and the mode of inheritance is polygenic [5]. The genetic basis of polycystic ovarian disease is supported by family studies that revealed that as much as 62% of the sisters of patients with polycystic ovarian disease will manifest polycystic ovarian syndrome [6], and 52% of the daughters of women with PCOD will manifest the disease [7]. The deregulation of the CYP11a gene has been linked to the development of PCOD. The insulin receptor gene on chromosome 19 is also implicated in the pathogenesis of PCOD [5]

Obesity has also been established as a risk factor, as polycystic ovarian disease is commoner in the obese population. Hyperandrogenism has been known to play a role in obese patients. The exact role that hyperandrogenism plays however has been poorly elucidated.

At the core of PCOD is insulin resistance, hyperinsulinaemia, hyperandrogenism, elevated luteinizing hormone, reduced sex hormone binding globulin and exclusion of other causes of hyperandrogenism related to ovarian and adrenal pathology [8].

AETIOPATHOGENESIS

The pathophysiology of PCOD involves several variables. There is a mix between environmental and genetic factors and variables peculiar to each individual. The final common pathway is dysfunction of the pituitary gland and development of hyperandrogenaemia. Folliculogenesis is disrupted due to the elevated levels of Anti-Müllerian Hormone (AMH). AMH demonstrates the best expression in small antral follicles. Low levels of AMH is fundamental to normal follicular development and normal fertility [9].

In PCOD, there is pituitary dysfunction that leads to elevated levels of luteinizing hormone. The pituitary dysfunction disrupts the pulsatile pattern of gonadotropin secretion. This disruption results in an increased secretion of luteinizing hormone relative to follicle stimulating hormone. This is what is believed to be responsible for alteration in the menstrual cycle tending towards oligomenorrhoea and amenorrhea [10].

Insulin resistance is defined as poor sensitivity of cells in the body to insulin, leading to increased circulation of glucose because the glucose in circulation is not being utilized by the body due to poor sensitivity [11]. Invariably, the body perceives this insulin resistance, as a lack of insulin and the pancreas compensates by producing more insulin, thereby creating hyperinsulinaemia [8, 12]. The state of hyperinsulinaemia that is created tends to suppress SHBG. A reduced SHBG means that the percentage of free testosterone available in the circulation is increased. The level of total testosterone may however remain normal.

Obesity is also related to elevated levels of testosterone. This is due to the peripheral conversion of oestrogen in the adipocytes of obese women to testosterone. There is also an increased level of dehydroepiandrosterone sulphate (DHEAS) [13]. In polycystic ovarian disease there is endothelial dysfunction and chronic inflammation. These create the basis for the development of cardiovascular disease and increased mortality later in life.

It is not clear if obesity as a manifestation of PCOD is a part of the symptom complex or a complication of the disease. PCOD and obesity can occur independently or they may be linked together. Insulin resistance is a common denominator between PCOD and obesity as both of these conditions are associated with insulin resistance [14].

There is a genetic basis for the trigger of an abnormally high androgen synthesis in ovarian tissue. A probable Mendelian pattern of inheritance has been put forward. Significant genetic defects could be transmitted to offspring in an autosomal dominant fashion, although with widely variable penetrance, dependent on several environmental and epigenetic factors, such as in-utero exposure to elevated levels of androgens [15]. Certain mutations in the genes of the androgen receptor, sex hormone binding globulin (SHBG), and steroidogenic enzymes could be significant in predisposing to the development of hyperandrogenemia.

Leptin

Leptin is an adipokine, a 167 amino acid peptide, that is secreted from white adipose tissue. Leptin has also been demonstrated in other sites including the ovary. The greater the adipose tissue, the greater the amount of leptin secreted. Leptin is either found free or circulating bound to leptin receptor. Leptin functions in energy haemostasis, reproduction and neuro endocrine function. Individuals with leptin deficiency suffer from infertility, underpinning the role of leptin in Fertility. This substance is thought to play a role in PCOD. In patients with PCOD there is hyperleptinaemia. In non obese patients, hyperleptinaemia have been demonstrated showing that hyperleptinaemia may not necessarily be linked only to adiposity [16]. Hyperleptinaemia has been shown to affect follicular development thus inhibiting ovulation [16].

Diagnostic Criteria

PCOD is a diagnosis of exclusion. Other causes of hyperandrogenism, hormonal imbalance and hirsutism should be excluded before a diagnosis of PCOD can be made [1, 17]. These conditions include adrenal dysfunction, thyroid dysfunction, hyperprolactinaemia and genetic conditions such as adult onset congenital adrenal hyperplasia. It is worthy of note that insulin resistance and disease conditions related to metabolic syndrome are not part of the diagnostic criteria. Further research may lead to evolution of the diagnostic criteria.

The highly heterogeneous nature of PCOD has made it necessary to develop diagnostic criteria for this condition. These diagnostic criteria ensure that standardized methods are used in making diagnosis and estimating true incidence and prevalence. The first set of diagnostic criteria were instituted by the National Institutes of Health (NIH) of the US in 1990 [18]. The NIH criteria include features of hyperandrogenism and chronic anovulation, without incorporating ultrasound features of polycystic ovary. Inclusion of ultrasound findings of polycystic ovaries tends to increase the prevalence of PCOD.

In 2004, the American Society of Reproductive Medicine (ASRM) and the European Society of Human Reproduction and Embryology (ESHRE) came up with a consensus on diagnostic criteria at the Rotterdam consensus. A patient is diagnosed as having polycystic ovarian syndrome, if demonstrating two out of the three defined features.

The features include:

- Amenorrhea/Anovulation
- Polycystic ovary
- Clinical and biochemical features of hyperandrogenism.

Clinical Features

The patients with polycystic ovarian disease could present to a broad range of clinical practitioners due to the highly heterogeneous pattern of manifestation. These patients could present to the gynaecologist, physician, endocrinologist, dermatologist or a clinical nurse. The patient's age of presentation and the nature of presentation will influence the clinician who will offer care to the patient. A young adult patient may present with irregular menstrual periods tending towards oligomenorrhoea and in some cases amenorrhea. Galactorrhoea may be present in some patients as well as hirsutism [19].

Patients with PCOD will manifest clinical features of ovarian dysfunction like anovulation and oligomenorrhoea or amenorrhea; insulin resistance and hyperinsulinaemia; features of hyperandrogenism such as hirsutism, acne and alopecia; as well as obesity, metabolic syndrome, recurrent miscarriages, endometrial hyperplasia, and infertility [20].

Menstrual irregularities: The menstrual irregularity seen in patients with PCOD could range from oligomenorrhoea, occasional menometrorrhagia to amenorrhea [21]. The basis of these menstrual abnormalities is linked to prolonged exposure to oestrogen not opposed by post-ovulatory progesterone leading to mitogenic stimulation of the endometrium. The labile nature of the endometrium leads to bleeding from the endometrium that is difficult to predict. However in some PCOD patients, the elevated levels of androgens could cancel out the effect of oestrogen leading to a thin endometrium.

Anovulation: Insulin resistance has been postulated as a possible reason for the anovulation as a substantial percentage of patients with PCOD treated with metformin demonstrated increase in pregnancy rates. Another factor implicated in anovulation is the large cohort of antral follicles inhibiting ovulation. This may explain the success in ovulation experienced when laparoscopic ovarian drilling is performed in patients with PCOD [22].

Hyperandrogenism: In PCOD, a state of chronic hyperandrogenism has been described that manifests as hirsutism, acne, with alopecia. It is of note that other features of hyperandrogenism such as clitoromegaly, increased muscle mass and deepening of the voice are not features of PCOD [23].

Hirsutism: PCOD is responsible for as much as 80% of cases of hirsutism. Other causes of hirsutism should however be excluded. The basis of hirsutism is elevated androgens. The interchange of androgens within the hair follicle plays an important role in this regard. Within the hair follicle, testosterone is converted by the enzyme 5 alpha reductase to dihydrotestosterone. Dihydrotestosterone is a more potent androgen and is more effective than testosterone in converting short soft vellus hair to more coarse terminal hair. This is more evident in the hairs in the androgen sensitive areas of the body such as the chin, upper lip, sideburns, chest and linea alba of the lower abdomen [24]. A scoring system has been developed to determine the severity of hirsutism.

Ferriman-Gallwey Hirsutism Scoring System: This method of determining severity of hirsutism is largely for research purposes. In this scoring modality, abnormal hair growth is scored in 9 areas of the body. Each area of the body is allotted a maximum score of 4. The higher the score, the more severe the degree of hirsutism. Hirsutism is described as a score of 8 and above. Racial and ethnic variables also play a role in defining hirsutism, as people of Mediterranean origin demonstrate a higher level of hair follicles than those of Northern European and Asiatic descent.

Ferriman-Gallwey Hirsutism

Acne: Acne vulgaris is a nonspecific feature of PCOD. Acne could be found in normal adolescent without PCOD. It has been demonstrated that women with persistent acne, are more likely to have polycystic ovaries on ultrasound. The relationship between acne and PCOD is such that as much as 50% of adolescents with PCOD have acne vulgaris to a moderate degree [25].

There is evidence to suggest that as much as 80% of individuals with moderate to severe acne have ultrasound features of polycystic ovaries. The basis of acne in patients with PCOD is that there is obstruction of the opening of the follicle by production of sebum, hyperkeratosis, overgrowth of the commensal by the name propionibacterium acnes and inflammatory changes [26]. Elevated levels of androgen have been documented in women with significant acne [27]. The excess level of androgen is responsible for stimulation of the pilosebaceous unit. This invariably leads to an overproduction of sebum. The end result is inflammation and comedone formation. Interventions planned for the management of acne should target these features in its pathophysiology.

At the level of the hair follicle the enzyme 5-alpha reductase converts testosterone to the active metabolite dihydrotestosterone. The enzyme consists of two sub-types 1 and 2. In aspects of the body affected by acne such as the face, the activity of type- 1, 5 -alpha reductase is more, leading to more production of dihydrotestosterone [28].

Alopecia: Alopecia is seen more as the manifestation in male sibs of females with PCOD. It may however be found rarely in patients with PCOD. Hair loss in these individuals has a slow progress. It could commence with diffuse thinning out at crown or there may be bitemporal recession [29]. It is important to exclude other chronic health conditions when individuals with PCOD develop alopecia.

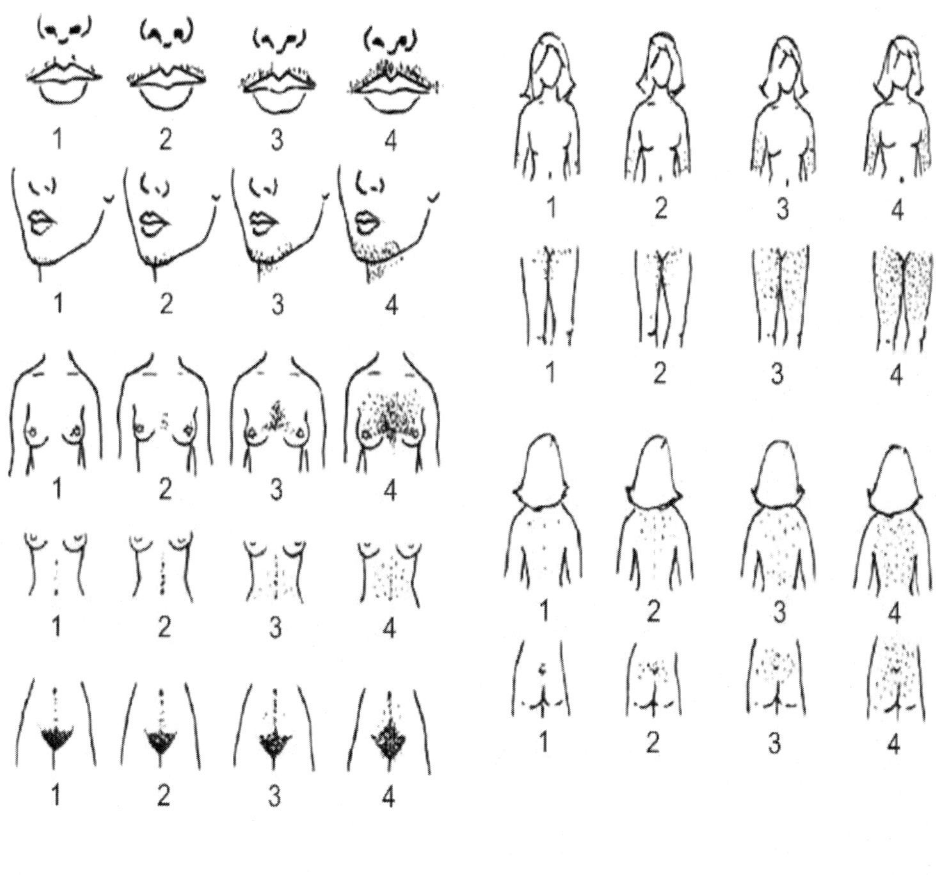

Onycholysis and Onychorrhexis: The finger and toe nails may be involved in some alterations in patients with PCOD. This could manifest in the form of onycholysis—separation of the nail plate from the nail bed due to involvement of the onychocorneal band, and onychorrhexis, splitting of nails in lengthway bridges. The relationship between this abnormality and excess androgen is poorly understood [30].

Acanthosis nigricans: This is a skin condition that occurs in the flexural aspect of the body such as the axillae, the groin, the back of the neck and the crease beneath the breast. The characteristic feature is that of velvety plaques that are thickened and gray-brown in colour [31].

Acanthosis nigricans has been viewed as a cutaenous manifestation of insulin resistance. However the condition can be seen manifest in individuals without PCOD. The basis of this skin manifestation is due to the setting of hyperinsulinaemia stimulating the keratinocytes and the growth of the fibroblast of the dermis leading to skin changes. The incidence of Acanthosis nigricans is commoner in obese patients with PCOD than in patients with PCOD with normal BMI.

Dyslipidaemia: In PCOD, there is elevated levels of total cholesterol, LDL, and triglycerides. The level of HDL is decreased and the ratio of total cholesterol to HDL is elevated. The implication of this is that the risk for cardiovascular disease is increased in individuals with PCOD [32].

Type 2 Diabetes Mellitus and Impaired Glucose Tolerance: Insulin resistance is the core of the basis of impaired glucose tolerance and DM in patients with PCOD [33]. This category of patients has been known to suffer from pancreatic B-cell dysfunction. The proportion of PCOD patients with impaired glucose tolerance is up to 30%.

Obstructive Sleep Apnoea (OSA): In patients with PCOD, there is increased risk of OSA. This increase in risk of OSA may be related to obesity but evidence tends to suggest that occurrence of OSA in patients with PCOD could be independent of obesity [34]. Obstructive sleep apnoea is a risk factor for cardiovascular disease in individuals with PCOD.

Metabolic Syndrome: In metabolic syndrome, there is insulin resistance, dyslipidaemia, hypertension and obesity. Metabolic syndrome is a strong risk factor for the development of diabetes Mellitus, of the type 2 variant and also a risk factor for the development of cardiovascular disease. The risk of myocardial infarction has been shown to be higher for patients with PCOD than in controls after correcting for other cofounders [35]. Echocardiographic features of women with PCOD have shown a greater degree of left ventricular dysfunction than in patients without PCOD.

Endometrial hyperplasia: The state of chronic anovulation in patients with PCOD creates a significant risk for endometrial hyperplasia. This is due to the unopposed action of oestrogen occasioned by the low levels of post-ovulatory progesterone [36]. This can give rise to endometrial hyperplasia and invariably endometrial carcinoma if not mitigated.

Infertility: PCOD is the commonest cause of anovulatory infertility accounting for as much as 80% of cases [37]. The disruption of pituitary and hypothalamic function affects regular menstrual cycle, causes anovulation and invariably infertility. This is usually one of the commonest reasons for presenting to the clinician. Infertility is a great source of distress to couples largely due to the great premium put on childbearing particularly in many parts of Sub-Saharan Africa.

Recurrent pregnancy loss: The rate of miscarriage in patients with PCOD is twice that of the general population [38]. The cause of miscarriage in this group of patients is poorly understood. A theory of excess LH secretion has been postulated. Efforts to target this excess secretion of LH has not been rewarding, thus dismissing this earlier theory.

Newer theories are considering insulin resistance as the basis for the miscarriage. Drugs used for the management of insulin resistance such as metformin, a biguanide has been used in some studies to manage early pregnancies in women with PCOD with some success [39]. Further well organised randomised controlled trials will be needed to further elucidate the role of metformin in the management of PCOD patients with recurrent miscarriage.

Pregnancy complication: Individuals with PCOD have been shown to suffer more pregnancy complications such as gestational hypertension, preterm birth and perinatal loses that are not related to multiple gestation [19].

Laboratory Features

The goal of laboratory Investigations will be to exclude other causes of hyperandrogenism, menstrual dysfunction and anovulation, PCOD being a diagnosis of exclusion.

Thyroid Function Test

Diseases of the thyroid gland can lead to menstrual irregularities seen in patients with PCOD; hence a thyroid function test will be required.

Prolactin Levels

Elevated prolactin levels, independent of PCOD can occur in women of the reproductive age leading to anovulation and infertility. This should be excluded as patients with PCOD also demonstrate elevated levels of the hormone prolactin.

Levels of Testosterone

Elevated androgens is a prime manifestation of PCOD, This is also a feature in late onset congenital adrenal hyperplasia, tumours of the adrenal gland and ovary. These conditions cause virilization unlike PCOD were features of virilization such as increased muscle mass, clitoromegaly, deepening of the voice, are not present.

In patients with causes of elevated testosterone other than PCOD, testosterone levels are quite high exceeding 200ng/ml in patients with ovarian tumours [40]. Imaging techniques such as ultrasound, CT and MRI are useful adjuncts to pick out ovarian tumours in cases of elevated testosterone levels.

Dehydroepiandrosterone Sulphate (DHEAS)

This substance is produced by the adrenal gland and elevated levels are highly suggestive of an adrenal tumour. Imaging techniques can corroborate the presence of an adrenal tumour.

Levels of LH and FSH

The gonadotropins show a variable pattern in patients with PCOD. Classically LH is known to show a two to three fold increase when compared with FSH in patients with PCOD. This does not occur always however; as some patients with PCOD will possess normal range of LH [41]. The estimation of the values of this hormone is also influenced by the use of Oral Contraceptive Pills (OCP), BMI, and the timing in the menstrual cycle.

Levels of Insulin

In patients with PCOD, there is resistance to insulin that invariably leads to compensatory hyperinsulinaemia. This is not yet considered as a diagnostic criterion for PCOD [3]. Determination of insulin resistance can be done via the following means:

1. Hyperinsulinaemic Euglycemic Clamp: This is the preferred method with better sensitivity, but it requires intravenous access, and is technically challenging. The same challenge applies to the Intravenous glucose tolerance test.
2. Intravenous Glucose Tolerance Test
3. Fating serum insulin level
4. Oral glucose tolerance test
5. Estimation of Serum glucose: Insulin ratio
6. Homeostasis model assessment of Insulin resistance (HOMAIR)
7. Quantitative Insulin sensitivity check (QUICKI)

Ultrasound

Pelvic ultrasonography is a useful adjunct for the diagnosis of PCOD. The route of ultrasound could be abdominal or vaginal. The vaginal route is preferred but a combination of both modalities is better than using one of them alone. Transvaginal sonography has a higher frequency and better resolution than the abdominal route and as such can detect features of polycystic ovaries better than the abdominal route. The wavelength of the transvaginal transducer is however shorter and structures that are far off from the transducer such as a huge abdominal pelvic mass coexisting with PCOD could be missed. This is the preference for a combination of both the transvaginal and the transabdominal modality of ultrasonography.

Ultrasound features of PCOD are as follows:

- Increase in ovarian volume greater than 10 cubic millilitres
- Small cysts numbering at least 12, measuring 6-8mm in dimension
- The cyst may be peripherally arranged in the format of "a black pearl necklace"
- Echo dense stroma
- This Ultrasound features must be distinguished from multicystic ovaries that exhibits fewer cyst, about 6-8 in number that are not peripherally located.

Endometrial Biopsy

Samples can be obtained from the endometrium of women who are more than 35years of age with abnormal uterine bleeding associated with PCOD. Endometrial samples can also be obtained from younger women with anovulatory bleeding, not responding to hormonal therapy

Differential Diagnosis

In establishing a diagnosis of PCOD, all of the possible differentials of PCOD must be excluded. A diagnosis of PCOD can only be made when other causes of hyperandrogenism, and or menstrual irregularities have been excluded. The following are the differential diagnosis of PCOD:

1. Congenital Adrenal Hyperplasia

This is an autosomal recessive condition involving partial or complete deficiency in one of the enzymes involved in the synthesis of cortisol and aldosterone. The enzyme deficiencies involved are 21-hydroxylase deficiency and 11-hydroxylase deficiency. 21-hydroxylase deficiency is more common [42].

In severe cases of congenital adrenal hyperplasia, manifestation occurs in the neonatal period with ambiguous genitalia and hypotension featuring in these neonates. The occurrence of hypotension results in life threatening consequences for the neonate. In this condition there is accumulation of 17-hydroxyprogesterone. This is a precursor of dehydroepiandrosterone, androsteindione and testosterone. Testosterone is responsible for virilization and creation of ambiguity in the genitalia.

Less severe variants of congenital adrenal hyperplasia may manifest features of hyperandrogenism in adult life.. This may mimic findings in polycystic ovarian disease.

2. Cushing's Syndrome

In Cushing's syndrome, there is excess secretion of glucocorticoids. These glucocorticoids could be exogenous or endogenous. The former is actually commoner. Patients with Cushing's syndrome manifest features of menstrual irregularities, acne, obesity, striae, glucose intolerance and dyslipidaemia.

Cushing's disease is a sub-set of Cushing's syndrome that involves excessive secretion of adrenocorticotrophic hormones from the pituitary gland. Manifestations are as expected from Cushing's syndrome.

Diagnosis is made from a 24 hour urine and estimation of the urinary levels of cortisol. A level beyond 300micrograms in 24 hour urine is suggestive of Cushing's syndrome [43]. An alternative mode of diagnosing Cushing's syndrome is to administer a dexamethasone suppression test involving offering to the patient 1mg of dexamethasone at 11pm and estimating the level of cortisol by 8.00am the following morning. Levels of cortisol above 5microgram per dl is suggestive of Cushing's syndrome [44].

3. Androgen Secreting Ovarian Tumour

In this condition, there is hyperandrogenism as reflected by elevated serum levels of total testosterone as reflected by values above 200ng/dl. In this condition, there may be no polycystic ovarian morphology on ultrasound and menstrual irregularities and anovulation may not be present.

4. Androgen Secreting Adrenal Tumour

This condition is characterized by elevated serum levels of dehydroepiandrosterone sulphate of greater than 700 micrograms per dl. Ultrasound features of polycystic ovaries may not be present.

5. Hypothyriodism

In this condition, there may be menstrual abnormalities, but there is absence of hyperandrogenism. There are no features of polycystic ovaries on ultrasound. Serum level of thyriod stimulating hormone is elevated. Neck changes may be observed in hypothyroidism.

6. Hyperthyriodism

The characteristic features of hyperthyroidism will be present, and this will include weight loss, tremors, proptosis, and in severe cases, features of cardiac failure will be present. Serum level of thyroid stimulating hormone is reduced. Menstrual irregularities and anvovulation may be present.

7. Hyperprolactinaemia

Isolated hyperprolactinaemia may occur in some patients with anovulation, oligomenorrhoea and in some instances amenorrhea. This should not be mistaken for hyperprolactinaemia that occurs as a manifestation of PCOD. In patients with isolated hyperprolactinaemia, serum levels of LH, FSH will be within the normal range. The level of androgen is also within the normal range and there are no ultrasound features of polycystic ovaries.

8. Premature Ovarian Failure

Cases of premature ovarian failure manifest with markedly elevated levels of FSH and also LH with very low levels of oestrogen. Oligomenorrhoea and amenorrhea are features of premature ovarian failure. There are no ultrasound features of polycystic ovaries in premature ovarian failure. Hyperandrogenism is also not a feature of Premature Ovarian Failure.

9. Hypogonadotrophic Hypogonadism

The characteristic feature is oligomenorrhoea, amenorrhea and anovulation with decreased serum levels of FSH, LH and oestradiol. There are no features of hyperandrogenism and no ultrasound features of polycystic ovaries.

Specific Interventions

The specific treatment intervention for the management of PCOD is tailored to the specific needs of the patient for the age group. The implication of this is that adolescents and young adults who present with menstrual irregularities are managed to rectify abnormalities of menstruation. Women who are planning or contemplating pregnancy presenting with features of infertility occasioned by anovulation will receive intervention to promote ovulation induction. Patients who along the line manifest features of Insulin resistance, diabetes mellitus, dyslipidaemia and metabolic syndrome will receive tailored treatments for these challenges. Hirsutism can be a nuisance for any age group and should be addressed. The following are the cadres of intervention that has been recommended:

1. No Intervention

In some individuals with PCOD, there may be enough menstrual cycles in a year and very mild degree of hyperandrogenism that negates the need for intervention. Women with PCOD who have more than 8 menstrual cycles in a year may not need any intervention to correct menstrual irregularities. Follow up of these women in the clinic is necessary to identify and manage features of dyslipidaemia and impaired glucose tolerance should these occur.

2. Exercise and Weight Loss

Exercise and dietary control are ways to attain weight loss. Weight loss as low as 5% of body weight, can lead to restoration of ovulation and fertility in some individuals. The weight loss will lead to a decrease in levels of insulin and androgens. All of these are initiated by an increase in SHBG [45]. A well balanced hypocaloric diet is suggested as the way to go. Diets high in carbohydrates tend to promote secretion of glucose and are thus not encouraged [46]. There is evidence to suggest that diet alone has beneficial effect in the management of patients with PCOD [47].

3. Management of Oligomenorrhoea and Anovulation Using Combination Oral Contraceptive Pills

This is the first line treatment for the management of oligomenorrhoea and anovulation. Combined oral contraceptive pills suppress gonadotrophins and invariably androgen secretion. Another mechanism for androgen reduction is via the oestrogen component of COC that increases the level of SHBG. Apart from the oral medication, combined oestrogen and progesterone can be used in the form of vaginal rings and patches.

4. Cyclic Progestins

This is used for the management of patients who are not suited for use of combined contraceptive pills. They are used to induce withdrawal bleeding every 1-3 months interval. Medroxyprogesterone acetate given at a dose of 5-10mg twice daily for about 12 days is recommended.

5. The Use of Insulin Sensitizing Agents

The classic insulin sensitizing agent is metformin. This agent used for the management of Diabetes Mellitus has found a place in the management of patients with PCOD. Metformin

has been known to promote ovulation induction, by reducing the levels of androgens [47]. Metformin is also known to reduce hepatic glucose secretion. Combination of metformin and clomiphene citrate has been shown to improve the conception rate of PCOD patients with anovulation [47]. Metformin, being a category B drug is safe to use as an agent of ovulation. Patients with recurrent miscarriages may find extended use of metformin beneficial in pregnancy.

The use of metformin for ovulation induction and pregnancy has not been approved by the FDA. When metformin is used for ovulation doses of 1500mg to 2000mg daily in divided doses with meals is the recommended.

The thiazolidinediones are newer agents used for the management of DM, with insulin sensitizing qualities. They are however category C drugs and should rarely be used as ovulation inducing agents. They should never be used in pregnancy.

6. Intervention for Hirsutism

The management of hirsutism involves lowering the levels of androgens. This will help to prevent the conversion of vellus hair to terminal hair. Hirsutism can be managed by medical means or mechanical means.

a. The medical agents are as follows:

- Combined Pills: The oestrogen component of the pill increases the level of SHBG. This will bind to testosterone and reduce the level of free testosterone.
- Gonadotropin –Releasing Hormone agonist: The agents act in a manner over time to lower levels of androgens. They create menopausal side effects such as bone loss and as such they are not good long term agents.
- Eflonithine hydrochloride: This topical agent is an irreversible inhibitor of ornithine decarboxylase. This enzyme is useful for hair follicle division and function. The inhibition of the enzyme slows down the growth of hair, but will have no effect on already established hair [48].
- Inhibitors of Androgens:

  These agents inhibit androgens and prevent hirsutism, but disturbing side effects such as metrorrhagia and ambiguous genitalia in male foetuses of mothers using the agent have limited their use [49]. When considered for use, they should be used in conjunction with oral contraceptive agents to take care of the side effect of metrorrhagia and prevent pregnancy. Agents such as spinorolactone, a diuretic agent are an example of an inhibitor of androgens. The potassium sparing effect does not allow its use with drugs such as angiotensin converting enzyme inhibitors, potassium supplements and NSAIDs
- 5 -alpha reductase inhibitors:

  5-alpha reductase is the enzyme responsible for the conversion of testosterone to dihydrotestosterone, a potent metabolite of testosterone. Inhibition of the enzymes prevents the formation of this potent androgen. This invariably leads to reduce growth of hair. Some studies have shown modest efficacy [50]. An example of a drug in this category is finasteride. This drug is also used for the management of cancer of the prostate

Mechanical methods of hair removal:

- Depilation: Hair removal above the skin surface. Shaving is the commonest method of depilation. It does not give rise to excess hair growth as suggested. Chemical agents for depilation are commercially available.
- Epilation: Removal of the whole hair shaft and root and involves methods such as waxing, plucking, electrolysis, threading, thermal destruction and laser removal.

Treatment of Acne

The treatment of acne is similar to treatment modalities used for the management of hirsutism. This is due to the fact that androgen reduction is the goal, and agents such as the combined contraceptive pills, anti-androgens and 5-alpha reductase inhibitors are of benefit.

- Antibiotics: Both topical and systemic antibiotics can be used. Systemic antibiotics such as doxycycline, erythromycin and minocycline. Erythromycin also has topical formulations as well as clindamycin
- Topical Benzoyl Peroxide:
  This drug has both anti-inflammatory and anti-microbial characteristics and it constitutes the active ingredient in many topical preparations used for the treatment of acne.
- Topical Retinoids:
  Agents obtained from Vitamin A that helps to maintain a normal status for the follicular keratinocytes. The agent possesses anti-inflammatory qualities. Many of these agents are category C drugs and are not recommended for use in pregnancy
- Isotretinoin:
  This agent is an analogue of Vitamin A. This agent should never be used in the first trimester of pregnancy, due to its teratogenic potentials. Its efficacy for the treatment of acne is however not in doubt.

Treatment of Acanthosis Nigricans

The goal of treatment in the management of acanthosis nigricans is to reduce insulin resistance, compensatory hyperinsulinaemia and excess androgen secretion. Insulin sensitizers will play a role in this regard. The use of topical antibiotics may be relevant in the management of acanthosis nigricans. Keratolytics have been attempted but there has been no significant benefit [51].

Surgical Means of Treating Anovulation

Attempts made in the past to perform wedge resection to promote ovulation in anovulation refractory to medical therapy are not as popular. This is due to the invasive nature of the procedure and the risk of the development of peri-ovarian and peri-tubal adhesions that can complicate further management of infertility. Laparoscopic ovarian drilling using 4watts in 4 aspects of the ovary has been suggested to replace the previous method of wedge resection [52].

In women not desirous of fertility, in very rare instances, oophorectomy has been suggested for women with severe hyperandrogenism and hyperthecosis

REFERENCES

[1] March, WA; Moore, VM; Willson, KJ; Phillips, DI; Norman, RJ; Davies, MJ. The prevalence of polycystic ovary syndrome in a community sample assessed under contrasting diagnostic criteria. *Hum Reprod*, 2010, 25, 544-551.

[2] Knochenhauer, ES; Key, TJ; Kahsar-Miller, M; Waggoner, W; Boots, LR; Azziz, R. Prevalence of the polycystic ovary syndrome in unselected black and white women of the southeastern United States: a prospective study. *J Clin Endocrinol Metab*, 1998, 83, 3078-3082.

[3] Rotterdam ESHRE/ASRM-Sponsored PCOS Consensus Workshop Group: Revised 2003 consensus on diagnostic criteria and long-term health risks related to polycystic ovary syndrome Society. *Fertil Steril*, 2004, 81, 19-25.

[4] Teede, H; Deeks, A; Moran, L. "Polycystic ovary syndrome: a complex condition with psychological, reproductive and metabolic manifestations that impacts on health across the lifespan," *BMC Medicine*, 2010, 8, article 41, 2010.

[5] Legro, RS; Strauss, JF. Molecular progress in infertility: polycystic ovary syndrome. *Fertil Steril*, 2002, 78, 569-576.

[6] Govind, A; Obhari, MS; Clayton, RN. Polycystic ovaries are inherited as an autosomal dominant trait: Analysis of 29 polycystic ovary syndrome and 10 control families. *J Clin Endocrinol Metab*, 84, 38, 1999.

[7] Yildiz, BO; Yarali, H; Oguz, H; et al. Glucose intolerance, insulin resistance and hyperandrogenaemia in first degree relatives of women with polycystic ovary syndrome. *J Clin Endocrinol Metab*, 88, 2031, 2003.

[8] Legro, RS; Castracane, VD; Kauffman, RP. Detecting insulin resistance in polycystic ovary syndrome: purposes and pitfalls. *Obstet Gynecol Surv*, 2004, 59, 141-154.

[9] Balen, AH; Conway, GS; Kaltsas, G; Techatrasak, K; Manning, PJ; West, C; Jacobs, HS. Polycystic ovary syndrome: the spectrum of the disorder in 1741 patients. *Hum Reprod*, 1995, 10, 2107-2111.

[10] Pellatt, L; Rice, S; Mason, HD. "Anti-Müllerian hormone and polycystic ovary syndrome: a mountain too high?" *Reproduction*, vol. 139, no. 5, pp. 825–833, 2010.

[11] Dunaif, A. Insulin resistance and the polycystic ovary syndrome:mechanisms and implications for pathogenensis. *Endocrine Rev*, 18, 774 1997.

[12] Doi, SA; Al-Zaid, M; Towers, PA; Scott, CJ; Al-Shoumer, KA. Ovarian steroids modulate neuroendocrine dysfunction in polycystic ovary syndrome. *J Endocrinol Invest*, 2005, 28, 882-892.

[13] Azziz, R; Carmina, E; Dewailly, D; Diamanti-Kandarakis, E; Escobar-Morreale, HF; Futterweit, W; Janssen, OE; Legro, RS; Norman, RJ; Taylor, AE; Witchel, SF.

Androgen Excess Society: Position statement: criteria for defining polycystic ovary syndrome as a predominantly hyperandrogenic syndrome: an Androgen Excess Society guideline. *J Clin Endocrinol Metab*, 2006, 91, 4237-4245.

[14] Dunaif, A; Segal, KR; Futterweit, W; Dobrjansky, A. Profound peripheral insulin resistance, independent of obesity, in polycystic ovary syndrome. *Diabetes*, 1989, 38, 1165-1174.

[15] Urbanek, M. "The genetics of the polycystic ovary syndrome," *Nature Clinical Practice Endocrinology and Metabolism*, vol. 3, no. 2, pp. 103–111, 2007. View at Publisher · View at Google Scholar.

[16] Martin, SS; Qasim, A; Reilly, MP. "Leptin resistance. A possible interface of inflammation and metabolism in obesity-related cardiovascular disease," *Journal of the American College of Cardiology*, vol. 52, no. 15, pp. 1201–1210, 2008.

[17] Azziz, R; Carmina, E; Dewailly, D; Diamanti-Kandarakis, E; Escobar-Morreale, HF; Futterweit, W; Janssen, OE; Legro, RS; Norman, RJ; Taylor, AE; Witchel, SF. Androgen Excess Society: Position statement: criteria for defining polycystic ovary syndrome as a predominantly hyperandrogenic syndrome: an Androgen Excess Society guideline. *J Clin Endocrinol Metab*, 2006, 91, 4237-4245.

[18] Zawadzki, J; Dunaif, A. Diagnostic criteria for polycystic ovary syndrome: towards a rational approach. In *Polycystic Ovary Syndrome Current Issues in Endocrinology and Metabolism*. Edited by Dunaif A, Givens J, Haseltine F, Marrian G. Boston, MA: Blackwell Scientific, 1992, 377-384.

[19] Boomsma, CM; Eijkemans, MJC; Huges, EG. A meta-analysis of pregnancy outcomes in women with polycystic ovary syndrome. *Human Reprod Update*, 12, 673, 2006.

[20] Apridonidze, T; Essah, PA; Iuorno, MJ; Nestler, JE. Prevalence and characteristics of the metabolic sydndrome in women with polycystic ovary syndrome. *J Clin Endocrinol Metab*, 2005, 90, 1929-1935.

[21] Coviello, AD; Legro, RS; Dunaif, A. Adolescent girls with polycystic ovary syndrome have an increased risk of the metabolic syndrome associated with increasing androgen levels independent of obesity and insulin resistance. *J Clin Endocrinol Metab*, 2006, 91, 492-497.

[22] Meyer, C; McGrath, BP; Teede, HJ. Overweight women with polycystic ovary syndrome have evidence of subclinical cardiovascular disease. *J Clin Endocrinol Metab*, 2005, 9, 5711-5716.

[23] Azziz, R; Carmina, E; Dewailly, D; Diamanti-Kandarakis, E; Escobar-Morreale, HF; Futterweit, W; Janssen, OE; Legro, RS; Norman, RJ; Taylor, AE; Witchel, SF. Task Force on the Phenotype of the Polycystic Ovary Syndrome of The Androgen Excess and PCOS Society: The Androgen Excess and PCOS Society criteria for the polycystic ovary syndrome: the complete task force report. *Fertil Steril*, 2009, 91, 456-488.

[24] Corbould, "Chronic testosterone treatment induces selective insulin resistance in subcutaneous adipocytes of women," *Journal of Endocrinology*, vol. 192, no. 3, pp. 585–594, 2007. View at Publisher · View at Google Scholar · View at Scopus.

[25] Dramusic, V; Rajan, U; Wong, YC; et al. *Adolescent Polycystic Ovarian Syndrome Ann NY Acad Sci*, 16, 194, 1997.

[26] Purdy, S; de Berker, D. Acne. *BMJ*, 333, 949, 2006.

[27] Bunker, CB; Newton, JA; Kilborn, J; et al. Most women with acne have polycystic ovaries. *Br J Dermatol*, 121, 675, 1989.

[28] Thiboutot, D. Acne: hormonal concepts and therapy. *Clin Dermatol*, 22, 419, 2004.

[29] Cela, E; Robertson, C; Rush, K; et al. Prevalence of polycystic ovaries in women with androgenic alopecia. *Eur J Endocrinol*, 2003, 149, 439.

[30] Özdemir, S; Özdemir, M; Görkemli, H; Kiyici, A; Bodur, S. "Specific dermatologic features of the polycystic ovary syndrome and its association with biochemical markers of the metabolic syndrome and hyperandrogenism," *Acta Obstetricia et Gynecologica Scandinavica*, 200, 89 (2) 199–204.

[31] Panindis, D; Skiadopoulos, S; Rousso, D; et al: Association of acanthosis nigricans with insulin resistance in patients with polycystic ovary syndrome. *Br J Dermatol*, 132, 936, 1995.

[32] Valkenburg, O; Steegers-Theunissen, RPM; Smedts, HPM; et al., "A more atherogenic serum lipoprotein profile is present in women with polycystic ovary syndrome: a case-control study," *Journal of Clinical Endocrinology and Metabolism*, vol. 93, no. 2, pp. 470–476, 2008. View at Publisher · View at Google Scholar · View at Scopus.

[33] Ehrmann, DA; Liljenquist, DR; Kasza, K; et al., "Prevalence and predictors of the metabolic syndrome in women with polycystic ovary syndrome," *Journal of Clinical Endocrinology and Metabolism*, vol. 91, no. 1, pp. 48–53, 2006. View at Publisher· View at Google Scholar· View at Scopus.

[34] Vgontzas, AN; Legro, RS; Bixler, EO; et al. Polycystic Ovary Syndrome is associated with obstructive sleep apnea and daytime sleepiness: role of Insulin resistance. *J Clin Endocrinol Metab*, 86, 517, 2001.

[35] Dahlgren, E; Janson, PO; Johnson, S; et al. Polycystic ovary syndrome and risk of myocardiac infarction. Evaluated from a risk factor model based on a prospective population study of women. *Acta Obstet Gynecol Scand*, 71, 599, 1992.

[36] Coulam, CB; Annegers, JF; Kranz, JS. Chronic anovulation Syndrome and associated neoplasia. *Obstet Gynecol.*, 61, 403, 1983.

[37] Hull, MG. Epidemiology Of Infertility and Polycystic Ovarian Disease:endocrinological and demographic studies. *Gynaecol Endocrinol*, 1, 235, 1987.

[38] Balen, AH; Tan, SL; MacDougall, J; et al. Miscarriage rates following in-vitro fertilization are increased in women with polycystic ovaries and reduced by pituitary desensitization with buserilin. *Hum Reprod*, 8, 959, 1993.

[39] Glueck, CJ; Philips, H; Cameron, D; et al. Continuing metformin throughout pregnancy in women with polycystic ovary syndrome appears to safely reduce first trimester spontaneous abortion: a pilot study. *Fertil Steril*, 75, 46 2001.

[40] Derksen, J; Nagesser, SK; Meinders, AE; et al. Identification of virilising adrenal tumours in hirsute women. *N Engl J Med*, 331, 968, 1994.

[41] Arroyo, A; Laughlin, GA; Morales, AJ; et al. Inappropriate gonadotropin secretion in polycystic ovary syndrome: influence of adiposity. *J Clin Endocrinol metab*, 82, 3728, 1997.

[42] Schorge. 2008. PCOS and Hyperandrogenism In Williams Gynaecology Eds Schorge et al.

[43] Kirk, LF; Jr. Hash, RB; Katner, HB; et al. Cushing's disease: clinical manifestations and diagnostic evaluation. *Am Fam Physician*, 62, 1119, 1133, 2000.

[44] Crapo, L. Cushing, s Syndrome: a review of diagnostic tests. *Metab Clin Exp*, 28, 955, 1979.

[45] Huber-Bucholz, MM; Carey, DG; Norman, RJ. Restoration of reproductive potential by lifestyle modificationin obese polycystic ovary syndrome: Role of insulin sensitivity and luteinizing hormone. *J Clin Endocrinol Metab*, 84, 1470, 1999.

[46] Bass, KM; Newschaffer Klag, MJ; et al. Plasma lipoprotein levels as predictor of cardiovascular death in women. *Arch Intern Med*, 153, 2209, 1993.

[47] Nestler, JE; Jakubowicz, DJ; Evans, WS; et al. Effects of metformin on spontaneous and clomiphene induced ovulation in the polycystic ovary syndrome. *N Engl J Med*, 338, 1876, 1998.

[48] Balfour, JA; McClellan, K. Topical eflornithine. *Am J Obstet Gynecol*, 194, 1266, 2006.

[49] Farquhar, C; Lee, O; Toomath, R; et al. Spironolactone versus placebo or in combination with steroids for hirsutism and/or acne. *Cochrane Database Syst Rev*, 4, CD000194, 2003.

[50] Moghetti, P; Castello, R; Magnani, CM; et al. clinical and hormonal effects of the 5-reductase inhibitor finasteride in idiopathic hirsutism. *J Clin Endocrinol Metab*, 79, 1115, 1994.

[51] Schwartz. (1994). *Acanthosis Nigricans: J Am Acad Dermatol*, 31, 1, 1994.

[52] Hendriks, ML; Ker, JC; Hompes, PG; et al. Why does ovarian surgery in PCOS help? Insight into the endocrine implications of ovarian surgery for ovulation Induction in Polycystic Ovarian Syndrome. *Hum Reprod Update*, 13(3), 249, 2007.

LIST OF CONTRIBUTORS

Dr. Endurance Ediriverere Aghahowa, BSc, MBBS, MSc (Physiology)
Research Fellow
Division of Clinical Sciences, Nigerian Institute of Medical Research,
Lagos, Nigeria

Dr. Leonard Ogbonna Ajah, MBBS, FWACS, FMCOG
Lecturer,
Departments of Obstetrics & Gynaecology, Faculty of Medical Sciences,
College of Medicine,
University of Nigeria, Enugu campus
Honorary Consultant Obstetrician & Gynaecologist,
University of Nigeria Teaching Hospital,
Ituku-Ozalla, Enugu, Nigeria

Dr. Getnet Yimer Ali, MD, MSc, PhD
Associate Professor, Consultant Medical Specialist (Pharmacology).
Director for Research and Technology Transfer
College of Health Sciences,
Addis Ababa University, Addis Abba, Ethiopia

Dr. Yifru Berhan, MD
Department of Obstetrics & Gynaecology,
School of Medicine, College of Medicine and Health Sciences,
Hawassa University Hawasa, Ethiopia

Dr. Cyril C. Dim, MSc (IntH), MSc (Phys), FWACS, FMCOG
Senior Lecturer,
Departments of Obstetrics & Gynaecology / Physiology,
Faculty of Medical Sciences, College of Medicine,
University of Nigeria, Enugu campus
Honorary Consultant Obstetrician & Gynaecologist,
University of Nigeria Teaching Hospital,
Ituku-Ozalla, Enugu, Nigeria

Dr. George Uchenna Eleje, MBBS, FMCOG, FWACS
Lecturer
Department of Obstetrics and Gynaecology,
Faculty of Medicine, College of Health Sciences,
Nnamdi Azikiwe University, Nnewi Campus, Nnewi Nigeria
Honorary Consultant Obstetrician & Gynaecologist,
Nnamdi Azikiwe University Teaching Hospital Nnewi, Nigeria

Dr. Oliver Chukwujekwu Ezechi, MBBS, MPA, MPH, PhD, FWACS, FMCOG, FRSPH
Deputy Director of Research and Consultant Obstetrician and Gynaecologist
Head, Division of Clinical Sciences,
Head, Maternal, Reproductive and Child Health research Group
Nigerian Institute of Medical Research Lagos, Nigeria

Dr. Preye Owen, Fiebai, MBBch, FWACS
Senior Lecturer
Department of Obstetrics & Gynaecology
Faculty of Clinical Sciences,
College of Health Sciences,
University of Port Harcourt, Port Harcourt Nigeria
Honorary Consultant Obstetrician & Gynaecologist,
University of Port Harcourt Teaching Hospital, Port Harcourt Nigeria

Dr. Titilola Abike Gbajabiamila, MBBS, MPH
Research Fellow
Division of Clinical Sciences,
Nigerian Institute of Medical Research Lagos, Nigeria

Dr. Megan E. Harrison, MD, FRCPC
Assistant Professor of Pediatrics,
University of Ottawa.
Division of Adolescent Medicine,
Children's Hospital of Eastern Ontario,
Ottawa, Canada.

Dr. Christian Chigozie Makwe, MBBS, MPH, FWACS, FMCOG
Lecturer
Department of Obstetrics and Gynaecology,
Faculty of Clinical Sciences,
College of Medicine, University of Lagos, Lagos
Honorary Consultant Obstetrician and Gynaecologist
Lagos University Teaching Hospital, Idi Araba Lagos Nigeria

Dr. Mark L. Norris, MD, FRCPC
Associate Professor of Pediatrics,
University of Ottawa,
Division of Adolescent Medicine,
Children's Hospital of Eastern Ontario,
Ottawa, Canada.

Dr. Victor O. Oboro, MBBS, FWACS, FMCOG
Professor and Head,
Department of Obstetrics and gynaecology, Ladoke Akintola University of Technology, Ogbomosho, Nigeria
Honorary Consultant Obstetrician & Gynaecologist
Ladoke Akintola University of Technology Teaching Hospital, Ogbomosho, Nigeria

Dr. Carol Odula, MBBS, MMed
Specialist Obstetrician and Gynaecologist
University of Kenya, Nairobi

Dr. Aigbe Gregory Ohihoin, MBBS, FWACS, FMCOG, DMAS, MCIArb (UK)
Chief Research Fellow/Consultant Obstetrician-Gynaecologist
Clinical Sciences Division, Nigerian Institute of Medical Research,
Yaba, Lagos

Ayodeji A Oluwole, MBBS, FWACS, FMCOG
Senior Lecturer
Department of Obstetrics & Gynaecology,
College of Medicine, Faculty of Clinical Sciences,
University of Lagos, Lagos
Honorary Consultant Obstetrician & Gynaecologist,
Lagos University Teaching Hospital, Idi-Araba, Lagos. Nigeria

Dr. Ngozi Clare Orazulike, MBBS, FWACS
Senior Lecturer
Department of Obstetrics & Gynaecology
Faculty of Clinical Sciences, College of Health Sciences,
University of Port Harcourt, Nigeria
Honorary Consultant Obstetrician & Gynaecologist,
University of Port Harcourt Teaching Hospital, Port Harcourt Nigeria

Dr. Tinuade Abimbola Oyebode
Senior lecturer
Department of Obstetrics and Gynaecology
University of Jos, Jos, Nigeria
Honorary Consultant Obstetrician and Gynaecologist,
Jos University Teaching Hospital, Jos Nigeria

Dr. Amy Robinson, MD, FRCPC
Assistant Professor of Pediatrics,
University of Ottawa.
Division of Adolescent Medicine,
Children's Hospital of Eastern Ontario,
Ottawa, Canada.

Mr. Alemayehu Toma, MSc
Lecturer,
Department of Pharmacology,
School of Medicine,
College of Medicine and Health Sciences,
Hawassa Univrsity, Hawassa, Ethiopia

Dr. Maryjoanne Chinyem Umeora, MBBS
Paediatric Resident
Department of Pediatrics,
Newark-Beth Israel Children's Hospital,
New Jersey, USA

Dr. Odidika Ugochukwu Joannes Umeora, MBBS, MSC, FWACS, FMCOG
Professor and Head,
Department of Obstetrics and Gynaecology,
Ebonyi State University
Abakaliki, Nigeria.
Honorary Consultant Obstetetician and Gynaecologist,
Federal Teaching Hospital,
Abakili ki, Nigeria

Dr. Agatha Eileen Wapmuk, MBBS, MPH
Research Fellow
Division of Clinical Sciences, Nigerian Institute of Medical Research,
Lagos, Nigeria

INDEX

#

A

B

C

D

E

F

G

H

I

J

K

L

M

N

O

P

Q

R

S

T

U

V

W

X

Y

Z